Dear, dear

Thank you for your
help — your encourage
ment and your love.

Fondly
Larry + Valerie

You Can Save Your Breast

You *Can* Save Your Breast

One Woman's Experience with Radiation Therapy

Larry and Valere Althouse

Foreword by
Luther W. Brady, M.D.

W · W · Norton & Company
New York London

Published simultaneously in Canada by George J. McLeod Limited, Toronto.
Printed in the United States of America.

Library of Congress Cataloging in Publication Data
Althouse, Larry.
You Can Save Your Breast
Bibliography: p.
Includes index.
1. Breast—Cancer—Radiotherapy. 2. Mastectomy.
3. Oncologists—Attitudes. I. Althouse, Valere, F.
II. Title.
RC280.B8A44 1982 616.99'4490642 81-18721
AACR2
ISBN 0-393-01507-6

W · W · Norton & Company, Inc. 500 Fifth Avenue,
New York, N. Y. 10110
W · W · Norton & Company Ltd. 37 Great Russell Street,
London WC1B 3NU

1 2 3 4 5 6 7 8 9 0

This book is dedicated to our parents:

Dennis Winston Fuller
Eula Cozart Fuller
Wilson K. Althouse
Kathleen E. Althouse

who in their different ways
prepared us for
and sustained us through
this life-changing experience.

Contents

Foreword

This is the story of one woman's struggle to exercise her right to participate in the decision relating to treatment for cancer of the breast.

With the discovery of a lump in her breast, she encountered the indifference of physicians, threats, warnings about wrong decisions, and scare stories. In large measure, the surgeons' recommendations were for radical mastectomy. Their views were limited and narrow, often unyielding in the demand that the breast be removed once the diagnosis of cancer had been established. Without exception, no surgeon she encountered would listen to her concerns, present the various alternative treatments, or even recommend that she see another physician who might be expert in discussing viable alternative treatment programs.

No physician is perfect—nor would the patient require the physician to be perfect—but, on the other hand, it is the responsibility and duty of every physician to be aware of the various alternatives in treatment programs and to present them fairly to the cancer patient, in order that an intelligent decision regarding treatment can be made.

Refusing to be intimidated, Valere Althouse came to me

at Hahnemann Hospital with an early Stage I breast cancer tumor. She and her husband chose treatment by radiation therapy, following the surgical removal of the lump. The result is excellent, not only from the standpoint of cure, but also she has a breast that is essentially indistinguishable from the opposite normal breast.

This woman and her husband have triumphed, over the opposition of her physicians, to achieve a program that was successful.

This is her story, her travail, her success.

Luther W. Brady, M.D.
Professor and Chairman
Department of Radiation Therapy and Nuclear Medicine
Hahnemann Medical College and Hospital
Philadelphia, Pennsylvania

Acknowledgments

This book is, of course, our own story. It represents our experiences—as we saw them—and our feelings and opinions about those experiences. Whatever errors in fact or judgment may be found in our story are solely ours as well.

Nevertheless, there are many people who, in one way or another, have contributed to that story and made possible the telling of it. We are deeply aware of our indebtedness for their encouragement and assistance. We cannot name them all, but we are particularly grateful to C.A. and Sylvia Rundell, Paul and Pat Fenske, and Martin Ebon, for encouraging us to write and attempt to publish this story, and for their respective efforts to help us; to Norman Cousins, who brought the manuscript to the attention of our publisher; to Dr. Samuel Madell who steered us to Mr. Cousins; to Irene Stuckey, who offered us the use of her house in Santa Fe so that we might complete the manuscript; to Carol Houck Smith, our editor at W. W. Norton, for believing in this project and providing us with her invaluable editorial help; to Dr. J. Robert McTammany and Dr. John R. Loughead, who not only gave us valuable counsel, but recommended that we get in touch with Dr. Luther W. Brady and his fine staff and Hahnemann Hospital. Having first of all encouraged us to believe that he could successfully treat Valere's cancer *and* save her breast, Dr. Brady consented to help us with this project by providing us with reams of technical materials, as well as numerous introductions and references to his medical colleagues. He also graciously agreed to read the manuscript. Without him, the story might have been a different one and this book would not have been written.

Finally, thanks be to God, who is in the midst of every healing and who, we believe, led us to the conviction that we should share our story with others.

"*Don't let them cut it off, Larry,*" said the familiar voice at the other end of the line. "*It's not necessary!*"

These words, spoken by a doctor-friend thirteen hundred miles away, saved Valere from losing a breast.

This book is written with the hope that it may do the same thing for countless others who are unaware of a relatively new treatment for victims of breast cancer.

You Can Save Your Breast

1. Almost Too Late

Few women are concerned with the possibility of losing a breast to cancer until that awful moment when a physician says, "I think we'd better get a biopsy; there's something there that bothers me."

We know, because Valere was one of those women.

No matter how unemotionally or even lightheartedly those words, "breast . . . biopsy," may be spoken, the patient invariably reacts with cold fear—at the very least. Unfortunately, by the time this happens it is usually too late to discover what every woman and many men ought to know about breast cancer: *it is no longer always necessary to lose a breast to cancer.* There is, in fact, a viable alternative to the traumatic and disfiguring surgery that is the standard treatment in most hospitals in the United States and many areas of the world.

Why is it usually too late? Because if a patient does not know that there is an alternative to breast surgery before she comes face to face with the surgeon, she is not likely to make that discovery once the chain of events leading to the operating room has begun. Numb with shock and fear, the patient may agree to both a surgical biopsy and mastectomy in one go-for-broke operation, simply because she does not realize that she has another choice.

It was almost too late for us. We came very close to making this mistake. We were unaware of any alternative to surgery and the two surgeons we consulted led us to believe that there was no choice other than radical surgery—the complete surgical removal of the breast. Fortunately for us, in the nick of time we discovered that there is another way.

Ignorance about breast cancer can be disastrous, if not fatal. Most of us are ignorant about breast cancer, and we are ignorant primarily because we choose to be ignorant. We don't know because we don't want to know. To be sure, the widely publicized radical mastectomies of Betty Ford and Happy Rockefeller did jolt the public into a new degree of awareness and concern. As a result, more and more women are now performing the regular and simple self-examination advocated so vigorously by the American Cancer Society and the medical establishment. But that comparatively small ripple of public enlightenment was scarcely enough.

What makes this particular ignorance so tragic is that once a mastectomy has been performed, it is irrevocable! You cannot reinstate the breast and try another form of therapy. Therefore, if you are among the 111,000 women who may be diagnosed as having breast cancer in 1982, it is vital that you learn some of the basic facts *now* and consider the current alternatives.

One out of thirteen women develop breast cancer sometime during their lives. We hope that you will not be one of these, but the possibility is not remote; breast cancer is anything but a rare disease. In fact, it is the most common form of cancer in women, accounting for 28 percent of all their malignancies.

If you are apparently healthy at this moment, it is understandable that you may not want to learn anything about breast cancer in general, let alone think of it in personal terms. Books and articles on the subject are not likely to be among your favorite reading materials. Perhaps you have never read anything about it beyond an occasional mention in newspapers and periodicals.

That's the way it was with us. We had virtually no knowledge about breast cancer and we had little interest in being informed. Why should we? Valere seemed a most unlikely candidate for it and I knew, of course, that breast cancer never occurs in men.

We were wrong on both counts!

We had assumed that breast cancer was most unlikely for Valere because, for one thing, there has never been any breast cancer in her family. Then, too, she has been blessed with excellent health, experiencing few colds (common or uncommon), coughs, viruses, or any of the other routine afflictions. She is an energetic, dynamic, and seemingly tireless woman in the middle years of life. Although she now finds it more difficult to maintain a constant weight, she still easily wears the same size eight she wore as a high school graduate. She eats a well-balanced and nutritious diet that includes the things nutritionists tell us we ought to have and excludes most of the things they say we ought not to have. She almost never touches alcohol and has never smoked. Both of us follow a daily program of calisthenics and walk three miles almost every day. Aside from a pituitary deficiency that has been kept in check for thirty years, Valere has generally regarded illness as something that happens to other people and breast cancer in particular as having no possible relevance for her.

Because her attitude is probably similar to many who read this book, we are using our own experience as an illustration. I say *we* because this is an issue with ramifications for both men and women. Some may choose to go it alone and others may have to, but if you are married, this is something to which both husband and wife will need to respond. It is also true that cancer of the breast is not limited to women, although admittedly the incidence in men is rare.

When breast cancer becomes a reality, it is a sudden intrusion that in a few short weeks can make a major difference in a woman's life, as well as the life of a family. That's the way it was for us.

One bright Dallas morning, Valere grimaced as we got out of bed.

"What's that for?" I wanted to know.

"Oh, I don't know," she said, making a wry face. "Something just doesn't feel right in my right breast."

"Do you have pain?" I asked.

"No—I can't say exactly what it feels like," she answered uncertainly. "It's more a pulling sensation. I must have slept in an awkward position."

The alien feeling was dismissed, and we began our daily routine. Later that evening, I asked her if her breast was still bothering her. She seemed hesitant to commit herself to a response.

"Well," I said, "if it's not any better by the end of the weekend, I think we should check it out with the doctor on Monday morning." And with that we both dismissed the subject again.

But it wouldn't stay dismissed and when Monday came, the sensation had not gone away as we expected it would. Valere called her gynecologist's office and asked the nurse to have the doctor call back. We didn't make an appointment because we half-assumed, half-hoped that he would say that it was not worth coming to the office.

Two days went by and the doctor did not return the call. Valere's breast continued to feel sore ("Not really sore," she would say, "but I don't know how else to describe it."), so she called the doctor's office again and again the nurse promised to have the doctor return the call. But he didn't, so on Friday morning Valere called a third time with the intention of speaking to no one but the doctor himself. This time, however, the nurse had a message for her: "Dr. Cromwell* said there's no need for you to see him until you get a mammogram." A mammogram, she explained, is a specialized X ray of the breasts and could be obtained at a nearby radiology laboratory. That same afternoon Valere made an appointment for her mammogram the following Tuesday.

The subject was hardly mentioned that weekend. The discomfort, we were certain, was nothing to cause concern and the mammogram was simply routine. We were somewhat annoyed that the gynecologist had taken so long to respond and then through his nurse, but we took that to indicate that he felt Valere's complaint was minor. Ironically, the discomfort in her breast seemed to go away during the weekend—or was it that the sensation was so slight that she was no longer aware of it?

The new week dawned brightly. The Dallas weather was perfect and we saw October get off to a good start at Texas Stadium with a Cowboys victory on the gridiron. The coming weekend promised a trip to Chicago for McDonald's hamburger magnate, Ray Kroc's seventieth birthday gala. Larry's new book was due in the bookstores that week. Valere's busy schedule included her weekly lecture to the women at the Greenhouse, the usual number of appointments, some club meetings, the arrival of our youngest son, Todd, to spend his fall break from college with us—and one mammogram sandwiched in among everything else.

Actually, *sandwich* is an appropriate term to associate with a mammogram. The process, as Betty Rollin describes it in her book *First You Cry,* is very much like making a "breast sandwich." The radiology technician, usually a woman, places the breast—yours!—on a cold slab of metal and lowers another metal slab until the

---

*Names marked with an asterisk have been changed by the authors.

breast is held firmly between them. The procedure is supposed to be a painless experience, but if the technician is careless or rough—Valere said hers was both—it can be uncomfortable and even painful. Fortunately the X-ray photos take only a few moments, although Valere had to repeat the process so that her left breast could be X-rayed as well. Apparently the gynecologist had ordered that both breasts be photographed as a routine measure.

Valere was soon back in the waiting room, presumably waiting until the technician was certain that the X rays were adequate. As she waited, she tried to read a magazine. Soon, however, she realized that she was reading the same paragraph over and over. Despite her confident self-assurance, it was obvious that a chilling fear had managed to slip through. "This is ridiculous," she told herself, "there is nothing to worry about." But even as she repeated that reassurance she was aware that her gut feeling was really something else.

At last, the technician, crisp and unsmiling, appeared at the doorway to inform Valere that she could leave.

"What about the results?" Valere wanted to know.

"They'll be mailed to your doctor tomorrow," replied the nurse.

"But we're going away this weekend," Valere protested, "and we want to know the results before we leave town."

Unmoved, the technician said, "We will mail them to your physician tomorrow," as she disappeared into the hallway and closed the door.

Apart from describing the experience to me, particularly the insensitivity and impersonality of it (hardly a rarity in medical care today, we learned), Valere said little about the mammogram as the week wore on. If we didn't hear from Dr. Cromwell by Friday morning, we had decided, we would call him.

This time we didn't have to wait that long. Thursday afternoon he called us. Explaining that Valere was out for a few hours, I asked: "What were the results of the mammogram?" In his voice there was a hesitation and reluctance that signaled bad news: "Well, the right breast seems O.K., probably just fibroid disease, benign, you understand?" There was another pause before he continued: "But, in the left breast—uh—there's a worrisome area—and I think you'd better get a biopsy."

"I see," I said without conviction.

The doctor seized the opportunity to end the call: "Tell Valere to call me when she gets in."

I'm sure we both said good-by, but I don't remember. I was stunned. Not only had Valere believed she was invulnerable to serious disease, but so had I. Of course, I knew that a biospy was necessary to determine if the "worrisome area" was really something about which to worry and I was sure that the report would indicate it to be benign. Still, I had not anticipated that we would have to go that far to prove it.

Suddenly I remembered Betty Ford and Happy Rockefeller and my mind leaped ahead: if worse came to worst—which, of course, it wouldn't—I would assure Valere that the loss of a breast wouldn't make any difference to *us.* We'd take it in our stride and our love would remain as secure as ever. But, of course, I reminded myself that I was wasting time in fruitless anticipation, because Valere's biopsy was bound to be benign.

It would be, I was sure—almost.

2.
A Worrisome Thing

Late that afternoon when Valere returned home I tried to be nonchalant as I recounted the phone calls that had come in her absence. I saved Dr. Cromwell's call until last: "Your gynecologist called and he said the mammogram is O.K. on the right side, but that there is something on the left breast that is, as he put it, 'worrisome.' He wants you to call him."

Valere's face fell and so did something inside of me. But we said nothing more, preferring to get the phone call over right away. This time we got through to Dr. Cromwell immediately and he repeated to Valere what he had told me, following with: "I think you'd better see a surgeon about a biopsy."

We both breathed a deep sigh as if for strength and Valere said, "But we don't know any surgeons: whom do you recommend?"

"Well," Cromwell replied, "I can't think of any offhand. Let me thumb through my directory here for a moment."

We waited for what seemed a very long time before he picked up the phone and gave us a name: Dr. Jowl*, "a fine surgeon," he assured us belatedly. We thanked him without meaning it and hung up. For a few minutes we sat and stared at each other before Valere said it for both of us: "Well, hell. I can't believe it! The *left* breast? They must have made a mistake; I haven't had any trouble on that side at all."

I acknowledged that I had heard of people's X rays getting mixed up and I recalled a newspaper article that told of a hospital being sued because they took out the wrong man's appendix. "Besides," I said, "a biopsy can prove either malignant or benign and yours is certainly going to be benign."

I called the surgeon's office to make an appointment for the following Tuesday. Suddenly, the weekend in Chicago didn't loom so brightly any more. The black cloud of "next Tuesday" hung over it and would not go away.

The next day a friend called and when I told her our disturbing news she was as shocked as we were.

"I can't believe it," she said. "But listen, I have just the right surgeon for her. He is the man who removed my benign cysts and you'll never find a nicer, more sympathetic surgeon than Dr. Moses*. Promise me you'll take Valere to see him. I know you'll love him."

Deciding that a good personal recommendation was better than Dr. Cromwell letting his fingers do the walking through the yellow pages, I agreed to call Dr. Moses' office to set up an appointment for Tuesday. So now we had two appointments with surgeons we hoped we'd never need: one with Dr. Jowl at 10 A.M. on Tuesday and one with Dr. Moses at 11. I decided to let Valere decide which of these we'd keep and which we'd cancel. But we never did get around to that decision over the weekend.

We did enjoy the trip to Chicago and the Kroc celebration was spectacular, but there was a heaviness that went with us and stayed with us. On Sunday, the morning after the party, we decided to treat ourselves to a lavish brunch in the top floor restaurant of the Continental Plaza. As I picked up my plate to start through the food line, an unbidden quotation bubbled up out of my unconscious: "The condemned man ate a hearty meal."

The weekend over, Monday dragged by. We still continued to ignore the need to cancel one of the appointments and when Tuesday dawned we had not even decided to decide. In the back of my mind, I suppose, I thought that if we liked Dr. Jowl well enough, we'd call Dr. Moses and cancel the second appointment.

Tuesday we arrived at Dr. Jowl's office a few minutes early and tried to read as we waited our turn. Before long the nurse summoned Valere, assuring me that she would come back for me after the examination. Dr. Jowl would be with Valere shortly.

Valere did not appear particularly nervous, but she must have been anything but calm and collected. In the examination room, she was instructed to remove her clothing from the waist up and then wait on the table. But when the doctor and the nurse returned they were shocked to find that Valere had undressed from the waist *down!* The doctor made a hasty exit while the nurse haughtily informed Valere of her error.

It was an amusing situation, but no one was amused. The doctor, it seemed, had probably never been amused at anything—perhaps he thought smiles were unscientific. When he returned, he got right to the task of the examination. He had seen the mammograms and his fingers probed the worrisome area on the left breast. He seemed to have some difficulty in finding it, however, and Valere couldn't help gasping with pain as his fingers poked and probed the soft flesh.

Apparently satisfied at last, he told her to dress and join him with me in his office. Valere has always been a quick-change artist, but on this particular day she must have broken all previous records. She hadn't liked the look on his face.

When we sat down in his office, he came right to the point. "There is a growth in the left breast that is a cause for concern. I have seen it on the mammogram and I have felt it in the examination. It's about the size of a dime and I do recommend a surgical biopsy."

He explained that a surgical biopsy means cutting out the tumor so that it can be tested for malignancy. This, he said, is done in two ways. First, while the surgeon and patient remain in the operating room, a small portion of the tumor is sent to the laboratory where the tissue can be frozen and examined under a microscope. If this indicates a malignancy, the entire breast is removed before the patient recovers from the anesthesia. The "frozen section," as he called it, takes only a few minutes and allows the surgeon to proceed with breast surgery without having to bring the patient back for a second operation.

The second examination is a more thorough examination of the tissue in the hospital laboratory and usually there is a wait of a day or so for a pathology report to be rendered, although almost always, he said, the pathology report simply confirms the verdict from the frozen section. (Later we would find that disagreement between these two reports is not so rare as we were led to believe.)

Bringing the conversation back from the general to the particular, I asked the surgeon if he thought Valere's lump was benign or malignant. I expected him to say something like "It's probably benign," but he didn't. Instead he said: "It's more likely to be malignant." Valere began to cry softly and I put my arm around her. The surgeon, I decided, might have made a good mechanic, but with people he was a zero. I was bothered by his matter-of-fact tone about something that could never be matter-of-fact for the patient.

As if he were uncomfortable with our emotions, he hurried on: "I have only one opening on my surgery schedule and that's Saturday—providing, of course, that we can get a bed in Baylor Hospital." We hardly knew what to say. We hadn't even adjusted to the idea of cancer and surgery, let alone to the possibility that we might not be able to get a surgeon even if we did accept it. So many momentous decisions to be made! We felt as though we were floundering in deep water while a sinister hand was offering us the last available life jackets. We looked at each other and I said what both of us must have been thinking: "Well, if that's the only time, we'll take it."

The doctor handed me a copy of a policy statement of the American Cancer Society. "Take this along home and read it," he suggested, "but return it to me. (I suppose he felt that for a mere fifty-dollar fee it was hardly worth his time to talk to us any further.) I glanced at it, but my eyes wouldn't focus, just as I was hardly hearing the doctor's bland, flat voice. He sounded like a sightseeing guide who had been on the job too long. He was saying something about "some people being deceived into thinking that they could get by with something less than a radical mastectomy." The paper, he said, would explain why the mastectomy was the only reasonable choice for a malignancy in the breast.

"But what about the right breast?" I suddenly remembered. "She never had any problem on the left side; it was only the right breast."

The surgeon was unshakable: "The worrisome area is on the left breast. There is no need for a biopsy of the right breast; that's just some fibroid disease."

Assuring us that his nurse would call us to let us know if she was successful in getting Valere a hospital room for the weekend, he dismissed us and we stumbled into the waiting room. There had been a finality about the way he spoke. The biopsy seemed merely a formality with him; he had already decided Valere had cancer.

As we waited for the elevator, Valere began to sob and I held her. People walked by without surprise or interest —suffering is the norm in a medical building. When we finally reached the car, I remembered the second appointment with Dr. Moses.

"What do you want to do?" I asked Valere. "Maybe it

would be good to get a second opinion."

Her eyes seemed focused on some far-off reality as she said: "But Dr. Jowl seemed so certain!"

"Maybe so," I replied, "but diagnoses have been wrong before and this one can be wrong too. I don't care if Jowl is a breast man (we had been told that he does nothing but operate on breasts); I'm sure he has been wrong a few times before and I'll bet he's wrong now."

So, because we were both still numb and still clinging to the hope that there was some mistake, we hurried to Dr. Moses' office just a block away. The waiting room was crowded and we took the last two seats. The nurse informed us that the doctor was running late in surgery but would be there very soon. "Very soon" dragged on interminably and I had all but decided to grab Valere's arm and steer her outside when the doctor arrived. At last our turn came and we were ushered into his office. We both agreed that we liked his style better than that of Jowl, who had met her for the first time under rather embarrassing circumstances on his examination table. Dr. Moses wanted first to meet us and talk with us briefly before examining Valere. Our friend had been quite right about him: we liked him immediately—although, as it later developed, not everlastingly.

Not having the mammography report, he asked more questions than Jowl had. At last he examined Valere, his face impassive as he gently probed the suspicious areas on both breasts. He was much more gentle in his technique than the other surgeon, another brownie point in his favor. Finally, he said, smiling: "Well, I think we ought to biopsy both breasts. There are mirror images on the two breasts." I vaguely remembered Dr. Jowl using the same terminology and guessed it meant that the areas in question were located at approximately the same place on the two breasts, although on opposite sides. Later this guess was confirmed.

"What's your impression from your examination?" we

asked almost in chorus.

"Well," Moses smiled, "I see more benign tumors than I do malignant ones." Our spirits lifted perceptibly. Some of our hope returned and we felt now that we had stumbled into the right decision in keeping the second appointment. Or had God pushed us?

Flipping open his appointment book, Dr. Moses studied it for a few moments before confessing that he had only one opening in the near future: the following Tuesday. There would be a convention in the city next week and with this one exception he wouldn't be scheduling any other surgery. Once again we were being offered the last life jacket and once again we took the bait. "Will there be any problem in getting a room at Baylor?" I asked, remembering Dr. Jowl's skepticism on that point. "None whatever," came Moses' confident reply.

This time as we walked to the car we felt we had been given some sort of reprieve. To be sure, everything still depended upon the biopsy itself, but Dr. Moses *had* said that he saw more benign than malignant tumors. That meant that he was going into it without expecting the worst, unlike Dr. Jowl. Our mood was mixed as we drove home, but at least we had some hope. We began to discuss what we would have to do before Valere entered the hospital in just one week. At least we would have a little longer to get ready: it would be Moses on Tuesday next instead of Jowl this Saturday. We were thankful for small favors.

That evening after supper we reviewed the day and the bewildering events of the last seven or eight days. We read the paper that Dr. Jowl had given us and I was surprised to find that all mastectomies required the removal of the whole breast. I had assumed that only a radical mastectomy took the entire breast. What Valere was facing, then, if the biopsy report indicated malignancy, was not simply the removal of the tumor itself, but the whole breast. The *radical* mastectomy, it seems, is distinguished from the *simple* and various types of *modified* ones by the amount of the surrounding nodes and muscle that are also removed.

Putting the paper down, I said suddenly: "There's got to be some other way!"

I was right, although I didn't know why.

3.
Is Mastectomy the Only Way?

Another way.

It was a conviction born of equal amounts of desperation and a lifelong optimism that any problem can be solved with sufficient amounts of hard work, clear thinking, and confident prayer. But it was one thing to say it and quite another to make that confession of faith a reality.

When I am not adequately informed about a particular subject, I try to find someone who is—someone whose knowledge and judgment I can trust. Among the names that quickly came to mind was that of Dr. C. Norman Shealy of LaCrosse, Wisconsin. He is a medical doctor, a surgeon who, as I remembered it, had given up the practice of surgery because he believed that much of the surgery practiced in the United States today is unnecessary and counterproductive. We had met at several gatherings where we were both on the program. Although I had not spent a great deal of time with him, I had found his ideas on wholistic medicine compelling and had been interested in the work he was doing at his LaCrosse Pain Clinic. He was a physician whose judgment, I felt, I could trust. When I called, his first words were, "I don't think I'd let them cut it off, Larry. I'm not up on all the alternatives to breast surgery, but I've heard some good things about what Samuel Hellman is doing with radiation in Boston. I'd look into that, if I were you. Many times the mastectomy is simply barbarous."

So there was the first piece of data to help us pursue our quest for some other way: a doctor named Hellman using radiology in Boston.

The second call I made was to a former parishioner in Reading, Pennsylvania, Dr. J. Robert McTammany. Bob and I had shared common ideals and convictions concerning health, disease, and healing and I had always admired his honesty and skill as a physician, as well as his spirituality as a human being. Within a few years after arriving in Reading, he had built a fine obstetrics and gynecology practice, which indicates that many other people shared my perception.

His response was almost word for word what Norman Shealy had told me: "Don't let them cut it off, Larry. It's not necessary!" And Bob McTammany took us a step further, saying, "I send all my cases of breast cancer to Dr. Luther Brady at Hahnemann Hospital in Philadelphia. He has had excellent results there with radiation, results as good as or better than what the surgeons are getting with the mastectomy."

Bob McTammany took precious moments from his busy practice to outline what the therapy entailed: a series of daily radiation treatments, and, in some cases, a seed implant. The word *radiation* stirred some unpleasant thoughts for I had seen too many parishioners sick and unhappy after radiation therapy. "What kind of side effects are there?" I asked.

"Almost none," was the reply I hadn't expected. "There's a burn of sorts—like a severe sunburn, you know—sometimes some nausea, but that's about it."

If I hadn't known that Bob wasn't the kind of doctor to minimize the truth, I would have assumed he was putting me on. "What about loss of hair?" I said accusingly.

"None," he replied, "not with breast irradiation."

Then I asked the question which, although I knew it was unnecessary, I had to ask just the same: "Bob, if this were Helen, what would you do?"

"I wouldn't have any hesitation in sending her to Dr. Brady," he said quickly.

For some reason I had to hear him say it just that way. It wasn't that I doubted his objectivity, but I knew that personalizing his advice with his own wife was the note I needed to hear. He suggested I call an associate, Dr. John Loughead, who had worked closely with Dr. Brady in Philadelphia. Loughead was happy to second Bob McTammany's recommendation and suggested I call Dr. Brady immediately.

"What about Dr. Samuel Hellman in Boston?" I wanted to know.

"Both Hellman and Brady use the same approach," Loughead answered, "I just know more about Brady's work because I worked with him for a while. He's a very fine doctor. You'll like him."

There was something reassuring in Dr. Brady's voice when I called him long distance. He reiterated all that McTammany and Loughead had told me and added more to the outline they had given me. "I know Dr. Moses," he said of our surgeon, "and you'll not need to come to Philadelphia until after we have determined if there is a malignancy."

Instead of a mastectomy, we were to instruct Dr. Moses to do a lumpectomy—a surgical removal of only the tumor plus about one centimemter of tissue around it. Before we ended our conversation, Dr. Brady gave us his home telephone number in case we needed to reach him and he wasn't at the hospital. Considering that we had had so much trouble reaching Valere's own Dr. Cromwell, that really impressed us.

So now we had found another way. The question that

faced us now was: is this the choice we need to make? The advice from Norman Shealy, Bob McTammany, and John Loughead, as well as the confident assurance of Dr. Brady, were very persuasive. Nevertheless, we remembered all too clearly the warning contained in Dr. Jowl's well-worn copy of the position paper of the American Cancer Society: radiation "has not been scientifically proven to be as effective as mastectomy." How to weigh four "birds in the bush" against "two in hand" and the prestige of the American Cancer Society! Obviously, we wanted to believe radiation was just as effective as mastectomy, but how could we be sure we weren't letting our emotions determine the choice?

The next day someone mentioned to Valere that a mutual acquaintance, Sally Lanker,* had gone to Boston to receive breast irradiation and had been immensely pleased with the results. Sally Lanker was happy to have Valere visit her and to share her experience. Given the same verdict and recommendations we had received from Doctors Jowl and Moses, the Lankers also had decided that there had to be some alternative to mastectomy.

Norman Lanker went about his research on breast cancer therapy with the same thoroughness and vitality with which he pursues his Dallas business interests. He contacted well-known physicians throughout the country and meticulously recorded and catalogued their responses. Although some of them knew of nothing beyond the mastectomy, several suggested that he pursue the possibility of radiation as an alternative to mastectomy. A few recommended that he contact Dr. Samuel Hellman at the Harvard Medical School Department of Radiation Therapy. Carefully weighing the data they had accumulated, the Lankers chose to go to Boston to see Dr. Hellman.

It was a decision they never regretted. The treatments were painless, the side effects were negligible, the cosmetic results on the breast were very favorable, and after two years Sally Lanker was apparently disease-free with both breasts intact. She showed Valere her breast and she was impressed with the results: not only had the breast been saved, but the breast was similar in appearance to its mate.

Sally urged us to go to Boston and Dr. Hellman. Sensing that Valere might need some further confirmation, however, she suggested that Valere visit another common acquaintance, Betty Leavell, who had recently been to Boston for Hellman's therapy. She also offered us copies of her husband's notes—forty-eight pages of handwritten notations. We were impressed: the Lankers had done their homework.

That evening both of us went to see Betty Leavell and her advice was the same as Sally Lanker's: go to Boston and Hellman. She described the therapy and her reactions to it, both of which were beginning to sound familiar to us. In addition to the daily treatments of radiation, Betty had also had a seed implant in her breast at the conclusion of the other treatments. The implant, she said, was like a booster dosage.

By the time we reached home that evening, we had decided to tell Dr. Moses that, if the biopsy proved to be malignant, we had chosen to receive radiation instead of the mastectomy. We also decided that Valere would go to Dr. Brady in Philadelphia rather than Dr. Hellman in Boston. Inasmuch as both doctors seemed to use the same methods and both were recognized in their field, it seemed that Philadelphia would be a wiser choice for us. We knew no one in Boston, and, Philadelphia was only an hour's drive from Reading, where my parents live. It would be far easier to stay with them than in a motel for five weeks. It would be good to have family around us during that trying time and, although we had not yet met him, we felt drawn to Dr. Luther Brady through our conversation with him on the phone, as well as the recommendations of Doctors McTammany and Loughead.

Valere had begun to keep a diary of her thoughts and

feelings, and she recorded the next day, Saturday, as a "pretty good day—kept my mind off what could be." We had a picnic with our son Todd and some friends before putting him on a plane to fly back to college. We saw him off at the airport knowing it had not been the "fun" visit we had intended it to be.

Saturday I also called Dr. Moses at his office and told him of our decision: if the biopsy proved malignant, we wanted a lumpectomy only and we would go to Philadelphia for radiation treatments with Dr. Brady. He acknowledged that he knew Dr. Brady and indicated that although he disapproved of our decision, he would do as we wished. I was greatly relieved for I had expected him to give us a hard time. My relief proved to be somewhat premature.

Sunday was a quiet day. The forthcoming biopsy shadowed everything we did, but we continued to hope and believe that the verdict would be "benign." Either way, benign or malignant, we were doing all that we could.

I continued to study the Lanker notes and a Xerox copy of a technical article which Betty Leavell had loaned us: "Radiation Therapy as Initial Treatment for Early Stage Cancer of the Breast without Mastectomy," presented to the American Cancer Society National Conference on Radiation Oncology, May 27–29, 1976 in San Francisco by Dr. Brady, Dr. Hellman, and eight other prominent radiologists. The paper presented data from four institutions: Hahnemann, Thomas Jefferson University, Yale University School of Medicine, and Harvard Joint Center for Radiation Therapy—a total of 150 cases. The results were impressive: the data for survival and tumor control showed that radiation was as effective or slightly better than mastectomy. Although granting that the study was based on a relatively small sample of patients and that there were some difficulties in comparing methods because of the nonrandom nature of case selection, different methods of staging, and different ways of reporting results, the report concluded: "We believe many if not most women can be spared mastectomy and the attendent emotional as well as physical scars." We couldn't help but note how this study contrasted glaringly with the policy statement of the American Cancer Society.

"Doing all we could" included prayer—a lot of it. We called friends across the country and asked them to hold Valere in prayer. Each day I gave her prayer healings and several times each day she used the visualization techniques which Fort Worth oncologist, Dr. O. Carl Simonton, had pioneered. We also asked for guidance: although we were certain we were making the right decision, we still asked for further confirmation of some kind. It had not been easy to make those decisions and I knew it would not be easy to stick with them in the face of pressure we might reasonably expect to encounter from those who would believe we were making a mistake.

Monday, October 17, dawned with its usual Dallas brightness. It seemed hardly an appropriate day for embarking upon so solemn an enterprise. We entered the admissions office of Baylor University Hospital with hope and fear. Admission was reasonably brief and upbeat. The hospital personnel seemed particularly helpful and friendly. Later, when Valere was established in her room, we were visited by Dr. Moses.

His visit began pleasantly enough. He hoped we'd change our minds about radiation and would consent to mastectomy if the biopsy proved to be malignant. Just as pleasantly we thanked him and reiterated our conviction that radiation was our best hope. Suddenly the pleasantries were over and Dr. Moses' approach turned to threats and intimidation. "Down through the years I've seen my fill of radiation patients," he said, "scarred, maimed for life—surely you don't want that?" It wasn't really a question, so he continued without waiting for an answer.

On and on he went, painting one gruesome picture after another. The more he talked, the angrier he became, the more insistent that we change our minds. We found it difficult to believe what we were seeing and hearing—the pleasant, cheerful Dr. Moses, now so hostile and unprofessional. Valere tried to tell him that she had seen the positive results of breast irradiation on her visits to Sally Lanker and Betty Leavell, but Moses brushed these aside with the intimation that they would regret their mistake.

At last, however, he seemed to realize that, although shaken, we had not caved in and, sighing heavily, he said, "O.K., if that's what you want." He told us that he would order another mammogram before surgery the next day, just to be certain. With that he said good-by, once again in a reasonably pleasant manner.

When I arrived at the hospital the next morning, Valere was in good spirits. She seemed positive and told me she was absolutely sure the biopsy would be benign. The second mammogram, however, had not been made and the nurse told us, when we inquired, that there had been no order for it from Dr. Moses.

The time to leave for the operating theater arrived and Valere got the best of send-offs, with friends there to see her off with me. I went to the elevator with her and kissed her as they got ready to take her upstairs. "I'll be right there with you," I promised and she knew what I meant.

As Valere was waiting to be wheeled into the operating room, Dr. Moses stopped to speak with her. "I think you're making a terrible mistake and I'd like you to change your mind," he said grimly. Valere simply shook her head no.

Now the waiting began. To take the edge off it I invited our friends to lunch with me in the hospital cafeteria. It turned out to be something less than the grand gesture I had intended it to be. When I got to the cashier, I found that I had left my money-clip and money at home. Our friends bailed me out.

Afterwards we went back to the room to wait. I don't know how long it was before Dr. Moses appeared in the doorway. He was still in his surgical gown. "According to the frozen section," he said, "the one on the left is malignant. Now, she's still up there and I can do a mastectomy if you'll agree to it."

"No," I answered wearily, "we haven't changed our minds."

"Do you realize what a risk you're taking with her life?" he demanded. "Do you want her maimed for life?"

I chose not to reply at all. I was getting angry and only my incredulity at his callous and unprofessional conduct kept me from exploding.

"O.K.," he said, "I cannot take responsibility for what happens to her and I'm going to write a statement to that effect for the record."

"You just do that," I said.

Valere's last thought before going under anesthesia was, "It's going to be all right." Her first awareness, as the anesthesia began to wear off, was of being wheeled into her room and seeing me ask our friends to leave us alone for a few minutes. "I knew then it was bad news," she says.

I can't remember the words I used. Probably I said what I had to say quite directly, for I could tell that Valere was already reading my face. As a pastor I had often been asked to deliver tragic news, but this would be the hardest of all those assignments.

We held and comforted each other. Valere was controlled, but understandably very sad. She remembers now that she faded in and out of consciousness, thinking, dreaming, and hoping. "I just couldn't have cancer," she had told herself. But she did.

It wasn't all bad news, however, for I told her that Dr. Moses had assured me that the tumor was Stage I (although at that time I hardly understood what that meant). It was very small and apparently had not spread to the surrounding tissue. It was the best news that she could receive and still have a cancerous tumor.

I called our friends into the room while I telephoned our daughter Tammy at the University of Arkansas and then my parents in Pennsylvania. We would be going up there sometime the following week to begin the treatments at Hahnemann with Dr. Brady. They assured us that they had plenty of room for us, as well as a car to use.

"It'll be more than five weeks," I told them.

"Well, we're sorry Valere has to go through this, but we're happy you're going to spend the time with us," they assured me.

I made one more call, this one to Valere's mother in Buffalo Springs, Texas. She is a woman of great spiritual faith, which was evident as I told her the results of the biopsy.

A loving family, concerned friends, and the prayers of so many people—we could feel the support from each.

I wrote a little poem for Valere. More than any gift, she has always treasured these stumbling attempts to communicate our love. As she read it, I could see she was deeply moved. In her daily notes she later wrote: "most of all he wrote me a poem of love that really made everything all right . . . almost."

The next day Dr. Moses came to see her. He was in a different mood, and seemed to be overflowing with confidence. After telling Valere all that he had told me about the tumor, he shocked us when he said: "I really don't think you're going to need that radiation; I believe we got it all."

Valere recovered more quickly than I: "Dr. Moses, yesterday you wanted to take off my whole breast as a 'matter of life and death,' and now today you're saying that you think you 'got it all' and I don't need any further therapy of any kind."

Undeterred by these apparent contradictions, he replied: "Well, it turned out to be considerably smaller than I first thought from the mammogram."—He had described it to us as the size of a dime—"It was only as big as a small pea. I'm really surprised," he confessed.

Valere, quick with her response once again, asked "Haven't you ever heard of prayer?"

We never saw Dr. Moses again.

Two days later when the stitches were to be removed, another physician did the work. Our only further contact with Dr. Moses was the bill he sent to us. We were satisfied to leave it at that.

At Dr. Brady's request, a liver scan and bone scan were scheduled, but for some reason they delayed the liver scan until just before Valere was to go home. So we had to go back to the hospital the following day for the bone scan and to collect the records we needed to take to Philadelphia for Dr. Brady. The hospital staff were dubious about entrusting records to a lay person, but at Dr. Brady's telephoned insistence they relented. We had a dinner party scheduled for that evening at our house but even if Valere had felt up to it, we would have called it off. We didn't feel much like celebrating.

The next day we packed and Valere wrote, "I was very sad and weepy." We didn't regret our decision, but it was traumatic to pick up and leave home for from five to seven weeks, not to mention the uncertainties of the therapy that lay before Valere. She seemed paralyzed with indecision: what to take, what to wear? I encouraged her to take absolutely everything she might possibly need. "I don't care how many suitcases you fill," I said.

We made it with four suitcases, one of them containing my IBM Selectric typewriter. The five weeks in Reading would not be a vacation. I would need to do lots of writing: my syndicated newspaper columns, a curriculum unit for the United Methodist Church, and some miscellaneous items that had piled up in the last few weeks. I was worried about carrying my typewriter in the small suitcase. I doubted it would fit under my seat, but I couldn't risk checking it through: it would never survive the journey.

Once again thoughtful friends made everything a bit easier for us. One of them brought by a splendid selection of fruit and cheese. When we arrived at the airport on Sunday, we found yet another expression of someone's love and concern. A Dallas friend had called American Airlines and upgraded our tickets to first class! I carried on my typewriter in its suitcase and it got V.I.P. treatment on board.

The Texas day was clear and beautiful as we lifted off from Dallas–Fort Worth Airport. It seemed we could see miles and miles ahead. But we wanted to be able to see even farther than that.

4.
What's a Hahnemann?

Before we left Dallas for Philadelphia we told one of our Dallas friends that we would be out of town for the next five weeks.

"Where are you going this time?" asked our friend, thinking we were off on another of our tours to some exotic corner of the globe.

"Hahnemann in Philadelphia," was our reply.

Our friend stared at us for a few moments. "Hahnemann? What's a Hahnemann?"

We gave an explanation that was becoming routine procedure in those few days before we left Dallas. Although Hahnemann is well known in medical circles and among lay people of the greater Philadelphia area, this fine medical school and teaching hospital has not gained the public image that has been identified with the Mayo Clinic, Menninger, or Johns Hopkins. I had known of it as the medical school where many, if not most, of the physicians in my hometown had received their education. I also vaguely remembered that at one time it had been a center for the teaching and practice of homeopathic medicine.

If we had been able to say that Valere was going to take her treatment at Harvard, the University of Pennsylvania, or Johns Hopkins, perhaps some of our friends would have felt more confident about our decision. Others were surprised that we were not going to M.B. Anderson Hospital in Houston, widely known throughout the Southwest as a hospital specializing in the treatment of cancer. We seriously considered it, for the therapy practiced by Dr. Brady and Dr. Hellman, as we understood it, is also available at Anderson. But we didn't have any personal recommendations for Anderson, as we did at Hahnemann, and besides we had already decided that, if possible, we didn't want to spend those five to seven weeks in a motel. Houston is just too far to commute to from Dallas.

We arrived at my parents' home near Reading, Pennsylvania on Sunday evening, October 24. At 8:30 A.M. the next morning we were at Hahnemann for our first appointment with Dr. Brady. We had liked what we had heard of him on the phone and we immediately found that he was every bit as gracious and friendly in person. It was not at all difficult to commit Valere to his care. We knew he was a physician in whom we could have complete confidence.

Dr. Brady took the better part of two hours to examine Valere and talk with us. He explained once again that Valere would come daily, Monday through Friday, for the next five weeks. The actual radiation treatment would take only a few minutes each day. At the end of the five weeks she would have received a total of twenty-five treatments, totaling 5,000 rads. At the completion of this five-week period, and after several days to a week or more to rest, she would be admitted as an inpatient for the seed implant of an additional 2,750 rads.

Then we were turned over to John Rowland, a clinical treatment planner dosimetrist,* who very carefully measured Valere and marked her for radiation. The purple

---

*A dosimetrist is a trained technician responsible for controlling the radiation dosage.

ink he used would be visible throughout the treatments and was very important for the technicians in directing the right amount of radiation to the right spot. Lead shields would also be used to make sure that radiation reached only the intended area. We were fortunate, he told us, that Hahnemann was using a new radiation device, a linear accelerator, which is more accurate and sophisticated than the cobalt machines still found in many hospitals.

We joked about the map Mr. Rowland had drawn on Valere, but beneath the joking there was a tension hard to dispel. No matter how confident we were, anxiety stayed with us much of the time. Only the friendly and concerned manner of all the people in the radiology department—Dr. Brady, Mr. Rowland, the nurses, the clerks, and attendants—kept that anxiety at a manageable level. A Polaroid photo was taken of Valere and posted so that she would be easily recognized by all members of the staff during the next five to seven weeks.

The next morning we drove again from Reading to Hahnemann, a drive of sixty to ninety minutes depending upon traffic. Valere was recognized immediately by the nurse who took her to the radiology room. As soon as she saw the linear accelerator machine, Valere remembered the dream she had had the night before she awoke with the discomfort in her right breast. In her dream she had been standing in front of a large and unfamiliar machine, receiving treatment of some kind to the upper portion of her body. She recognized the machine in the dream as the linear accelerator she now faced in the radiology room!

Many times in her life Valere has previewed future events in her dreams. Usually we recognize and understand the event she has previewed. But this dream, because we could not relate it to anything she was currently experiencing, had been forgotten. We can only conclude that her unconscious mind knew about her breast cancer and the treatment she would choose—before we even knew there was a tumor.

The treatment itself required only three minutes and, combined with the time in the waitingroom, took only fifteen minutes out of our daily weekday schedule—plus, of course, our commuting time. Before returning to Reading that day we clocked off a mile and a half on our car speedometer, beginning at the hospital and continuing to a motel that lay along our daily route. Since we generally walk three miles a day, we decided to park the car at the motel each day so that we might still get in our walk. With the exception of a few days when it rained, we maintained our routine throughout the five weeks.

Our daily trip to Hahnemann took the best part of the morning, getting us back to Reading by noontime. After lunch both of us worked: I at my typewriter and Valere with her lectures, workshops, and correspondence. Our weekends would be free, so we decided to make the most of the opportunity to visit friends and to sightsee. One weekend we went to Cape Cod to visit friends, with a swing around Boston to see its historical sights, stopping at West Point and the U.S. Military Academy on our way back to Philadelphia. Another weekend was spent in New York City, Connecticut, and Long Island visiting friends. On another I was asked to lecture in Harrisburg, Pennsylvania, pinch-hitting for a speaker who had to cancel at the last minute. We planned also to take one weekend to see Williamsburg, Jamestown, and Yorktown, Virginia, but a bout of flu caused us to cancel that weekend's plans.

One of the first physical reactions Valere began to experience was actually quite unrelated to the treatments. For sixteen years, as directed by her OB/GYN doctor, Valere had been taking daily dosages of hormones.* One of Dr.

---

*This prescription was given to Valere, not for any particular condition except that her physician believed hormone supplements were beneficial to most women, particularly in retarding the effects of the aging process.

Brady's first requests when she checked into Hahnemann was that she discontinue the hormones. Although there is, at this writing, no definite proof that hormones increase the risk of cancer, many physicians are sufficiently suspicious to make it a rule of thumb that all hormones be discontinued when the patient is diagnosed with a malignancy. The immediate result for Valere was the onset of severe hot and cold flashes. These were exhausting and extremely uncomfortable. So it is difficult to know whether the fatigue she experienced during her radiation was entirely due to the radiation itself, or in part to being taken off the hormones.

Another factor which made it difficult to assess how the radiation was affecting her was her *diabetes insipidus,* a condition she has had for twenty-five years. Unlike the more common *diabetes mellitus,* this rather rare disease is tied to the function of the posterior portion of the pituitary gland and its chief effect in her body is the irregularity of water retention and elimination, as well as thirst control. When her pituitary gland is not functioning correctly, she becomes extremely thirsty and cannot retain fluids. At the same time her body feels weak, tired, and sometimes a bit "trembly." The only recourse at these times is an injection of extract from animal pituitary glands, *pitressin tannate*—usually on a daily basis. Normally, after she has had her injection it takes several hours before she is feeling normal. Therefore during the five weeks at Hahnemann and in the months that followed the treatment, it was sometimes difficult to attribute fatigue to radiation, *diabetes insipidus,* or hormonal factors.

For example, in her daily diary entry for October 27, the second day of the irradiation treatments, Valere wrote:

> *October 27*—I felt slightly nauseated as we drove to Philly. I need a petressin tannate injection—badly. . . . It took three tries for me to get the needle in and a long time to take effect.

There were also some emotional factors at work. It was frightening to be shut up alone in the room with the linear accelerator and see the technicians safely shielded outside. Of course, this precaution was logical: Valere would be before the machine a few minutes each day, whereas the technicians were working with it eight hours a day, five days a week, year in and year out. Still, logic had to wrestle with the instinctive fears.

If I made a mistake during this period, it was in not fully understanding how exhausting the procedure could be. I reasoned that the treatment took only a few minutes each day; certainly that should leave lots of energy for other activities. What I failed to take into consideration was the ever-present emotional strain of dealing with the reality of cancer, the understandable fear of being subjected to a huge, powerful machine, the daily drive to and from Philadelphia, and living out of suitcases several thousand miles from home. Consequently, we scheduled too many activities and Valere disciplined herself to work too hard each day until we finally realized just how tired she really was. We also failed to take into consideration that she was recuperating from surgery, a considerable shock to both body and psyche.

So on that second day of treatment, following the visit to Hahnemann, we stopped by the Philadelphia office of Swissair to see some old friends and associates in the travel business. Instead of the quick "hello" we had intended, we wound up going to lunch with them. For me it was a pleasurable experience—I love travel in general and Swissair and our friends in particular—so I failed to realize what an endurance trial it was for Valere:

> I was limp, listless, and sleepy at Swissair and even more so at the sidewalk cafe for lunch. . . . I'm afraid I wasn't with it today."

The next day was Friday and we had planned to take off for Cape Cod immediately following the treatment at the hospital:

October 28—I feel better than yesterday. After the treatment, we walked back to our car a mile and a half away and left for Cape Cod. . . . I slept most of the way. . . . I was very relaxed but so hot, Hot, HOT! . . . I vaguely remember walking around Yale's lovely campus at New Haven. . . . Physically, it was a day of ups and downs.

October 29—While at Cape Cod I took no Belergal,* so I wasn't sleepy as I had been, but I was so hot. . . . The surgical incision on my right breast drained almost constantly over the weekend.

October 30—I tire so easily, and am so exhausted by night. . . . I get those awful panicky sweats—so hot! . . . I do so thank God for Larry's sense of humor and that he gets me into a different environment on the weekends. . . . As we drive, Larry and I talk and talk: what, when, and why did I get my tumor? According to people in psychosomatics, I created it or at least in some way I let it happen; so now I must take command of the situation. We listened to the Carl Simonton tapes as we drove—very good.

October 31—Back to Philadelphia to see Dr. Brady . . . He said I am doing O.K. . . . My left breast has drained plentifully all weekend, but he was not concerned. The draining, of course, is from the surgery, not the radiation. I told him of some slight pain in my ribs and he suggested that, if it should continue, I might try going without a bra. I did, but it was too painful as I bounced in the car.

November 1—Today I rode to Philadelphia with Gladys, another of Dr. Brady's patients from the Reading area. I'm embarrassed that I slept most of the way while she talked. She says she has no soreness or anything—so why do I feel

*Belergal is a prescription drug given to control heat flashes.

so bad? I take two Belergals per day—one at night and one in the morning—but I still get those awful *hots!* . . . I made myself do some work this afternoon.

November 2—No Belergal this morning, so I didn't get so sleepy on the way to Philadelphia, but I had those awful, panicky sweats. On the way down, Gladys talked of nothing but food and what she was cooking for her family. I felt so sick I thought I'd vomit all the way to Philly. . . . My neck and shoulders ache and I have a strange feeling in my head.

November 3—I must have a virus. I ache all over, especially my head and spine, and all the way to my lower back. I had a terrible night, but so did Larry. While at Hahneman, I asked Dr. Chen about it, but he assured me it was unrelated to the radiation. He must be right, for tonight all four of us —Larry, his parents, and I—feel sick.

November 5—Larry made an appointment for me with Dr. Bob McTammany. In his office I had a temperature, but he found nothing else. It was a good visit with Bob; he encouraged us to write a book about this experience so that other women can know. I felt better just knowing that nothing serious was wrong with me: just a 'bug' and everyone in the family has it—the family that stays together may get sick together! . . . It is hard to swallow; I feel as if there's a lump in my throat, like a plum. . . . So sore, but that's one of the reactions they told me I might have.

November 7—Back to Philly for my ninth treatment. Dr. Brady says I am doing fine, but now the plum in my throat is the size of a golfball, hard to swallow.

November 8—Eleventh treatment: slightly nauseated. . . . Bigger golf ball on left side of my throat . . . blue pills for nausea.

November 10—I feel much better. . . . Even got my hair done!

November 11—Good day. . . . Oh, slightly nauseated, but TGIF!

November 14—Dr. Brady says I'm still doing fine: no burn or infection in the radiated area. My throat still feels awful, more like a bunch of grapes—red hot grapes. *Hurts!* . . . Tonight I feel depressed. Why? . . . My throat is at its worst; it hurt all night and I slept little.

November 15—Surprise, surprise: I feel good!

November 16—Throat still hurts, but I feel good just the same.

November 17–21—Good, bad, in-between: itching on the breast began today and the throat still hurts.

November 23—Today there is some burning . . . deep red . . . itching . . . using cream—it helps.

November 24—Thanksgiving Day: a good one! Lots for which to be thankful. I have both breasts and I am convinced the therapy is the right course of action. Mother and Dad Althouse have been so good to us. That makes it easier.

November 25—Dr. Brady gave me a new salve to try. It's called Kenalog Cream. It's by prescription only and expensive. I've been using cornstarch and that has worked pretty well. He also told me to use Nupercainal Cream (sold over the counter) and keep my breast plastered with it.

November 26—I itch like crazy and yet I am quite burned. It hurts and is a little raw, so I can't scratch. He doesn't want the skin broken so that in a couple of weeks the thick, tanned, burned skin will simply lift off—he hopes.

November 28—Now I'm very burned. . . . raw and itching, even though I keep it covered with cream all the time. Dr. Brady gave me gauze pads to keep on it at all times.

November 30—My last treatment! Yay! Saw Gladys and she is now having some problems, too: infection. I'm thankful for my olive skin and the lubrication I've been giving it. Dr. Brady says it's O.K. to go home to Dallas until December 12—ten glorious days!

December 6—We're doing too much, but I don't want to miss anything . . . like the Bloom's annual Christmas dinner dance at the Dallas Country Club—it's always such fun. We came home early, but we enjoyed the dinner and had a few dances. I wore a dress with some cleavage—you bet, I wanted them to know.

December 7—This was a tough day: I felt so weak, no energy, my lung hurts, my chest hurts, and I am short of breath—sort of gasping. Otherwise. . . .

December 8—Started wearing a bra* again, but it's so uncomfortable. So I tried another that was too large for me—still hurts.

December 9–10—Good and bad. . . . Tire very easily. . . . Now my skin is peeling in sheets, just like Dr. Brady said it would.

December 12—Time to return to Pennsylvania—so soon. We fly back and once again I'm feeling tired, even though I take a nap every afternoon.

December 13—Checked into Hahnemann. . . . I felt almost drugged, I was so tired and sleepy. I could hardly talk and couldn't think at all.

December 14—Routine tests, i.e., urine, blood, X rays, EKG. Then to Dr. Brady for the implants. Larry watched the whole procedure so that he'd be able to write about it. It really wasn't bad at all, no pain, no discomfort. The implant,** they say, is an 'insurance dosage,' allowing them to

---

*Although during the first four weeks of treatment I needed the support of a bra, during the last week the skin became too tender and I had to stop wearing it altogether.

**The seed implant—sometimes inaccurately called a "needle" implant—consists of narrow nylon tubing with tiny iridium-192 radioactive particles. The tubing is sutured (stitched) into the breast tissue under local anesthesia. When the tissue has been exposed to the prescribed number of rads—usually requiring two or three days—the tube with the seeds is removed. Dr. Luther Brady believes that the use of the implant has, in his staff's experience at Hahnemann Hospital, eliminated the local recurrence of breast cancer.

deliver a high amount of radiation to a very limited area, more limited than what they can do with the linear accelerator. When they take me back to my room, I will be in isolation until the needles are removed. No visitors may come in the room, no closer than the doorway; dishes, linens must remain there.

December 15—I sleep a lot, feel drowsy . . . lonely. Larry visits each day—from the doorway.

December 17—I'm doing lots of meditation, thinking, and praying. I'm so thankful for Larry, his love, and his wisdom that brought us here. I'm also thankful for all of the gifts of love, concern, and prayer from so many friends. Isolation for four days and nights is hard, but Dr. Brady and his staff are so *nice* in every way. This morning Dr. Damsker and Dr. Chan came by and checked me, made me more comfortable with ace bandages around both breasts. I made myself stay out of bed in order to get more strength. The room is so small: I have walked it a jillion times, listened to tapes, read, thought, wrote out my own relaxation tapes, and given some thought to some other tapes I'll make for other women who have to go through this . . . tapes for isolation . . . tapes for radiation . . . teaching them how to use positive thoughts as they go into each radiation treatment.

December 18—Back to Dallas and home! It's over—oh, not entirely: I remain tired, achey, short of breath, etc., but I'm finding that each day I feel a little better.

In the months that followed, I made sure that Valere would take a nap every afternoon. It's hard to keep her from overdoing and overworking, so I had to insist that she set aside a rest period every day. The achiness and shortness of breath soon went away, but the fatigue took much longer to go away completely.

5.
One-Step vs. Two-Step Procedures

Valere was saved from an unnecessary mastectomy because we were fortunate enough to learn that she could choose among several alternatives. We have since discovered that many women have not been so fortunate. No one has told them that there are alternatives to the mastectomy; still less has anyone helped them to understand that they have a right to make that choice for themselves.

This book was written because we believe that *every woman has a right to know what alternatives are available in the treatment of breast cancer.* And that *every woman has a right to make an informed choice for herself.*

Still, before she can make such a choice, she needs to have at least a mimimal understanding of the normal and abnormal physiology of the female breast. The following information is admittedly much simplified. Readers may also want to consult chapters three and four of an excellent book, *The Breast* by Dr. Oliver Cope.

About Lumps in the Breast

We tend to think of the breast as a rather uncomplicated and fairly static part of the female anatomy. Once a woman has reached physical maturity, we assume that the breast remains the same size and shape until it undergoes the normal shrinkage and changes brought about by advancing age. The fact is, however, that the breast is quite complicated and anything but static. Change, growth, swelling, and shrinkage are constantly taking place in the female breast.

Because it is an integral part of the female reproductive system, the breast grows throughout pregnancy so that it may be ready to nurse the newborn child. But when it is no longer needed for that purpose, it begins to recede and to wait for another pregnancy, when it will start growing and swelling once again.

Actually, the breast doesn't simply wait for a pregnancy. Like the uterus, it makes a monthly preparation in harmony with the menstrual cycle. There is, in fact, a close relationship between the fibrous tissue of the breast and the muscle tissue of the wall of the uterus. Both grow and develop during pregnancy, responding to the very same ovarian hormones. Both swell with an increase in blood during the menstrual cycle. Unlike the uterus, which quickly gets rid of its pregnancy preparations through menstruation, the breast must absorb these excess cells that build up each month in anticipation of pregnancy. These excess cells may be experienced as a lumpiness in the breast. The accumulation of fluids into cysts may also cause the same sensation. This lumpiness is most noticeable as women approach menstruation in the months from December to May—the season when the ovaries are at peak activity—and disappearing thereafter. Women who detect these swellings of the breast often are fearful that the swellings or lumps mean breast cancer.

However, they may simply be the normal swellings that occur during the menstrual cycle.

Of course, other growths can occur in the breast. But the most common growths in female breasts are *not* cancerous. Half the women in the United States will experience fibrocystic tumors sometime in their lives. Although these tumor growths do require medical attention, they are not cancerous and the growths will either eventually disappear or may be removed surgically. At this time, physicians generally agree that fibroid tumors do not later change into malignant growths. Often they are removed surgically, not because their removal will prevent them from being cancerous at a later time, but simply for the comfort of the patient.

So let us understand that there is a lot of growth and change normally taking place within the healthy breast. Lumps in the breast do not necessarily mean breast cancer and finding a lump there should not cause panic, although further examination and watchfulness are justified.

About Cancerous Growths

As previously noted, 50 percent of the women in the United States will experience fibrous—and essentially harmless—growths in their breasts at some time in their lives. These growths are called *benign.* By comparison, only 7 percent of American women will develop cancerous or *malignant* tumors. What is the difference between the benign and malignant growth in the breast?

To put it as simply as possible, a benign growth is one which does not invade the tissues around it. These growths cause no trouble in the breast, except to exert some pressure on the surrounding area. They are abnormal cells, but they do not attack anything, although they may grow from the size of a small grape to a large plum.

The malignant cell, however, differs in that it not only grows, but it invades the tissues of the breast in unbridled growth and may reach remote parts of the body. When this happens, it is said that the growth has *metastasized.* A benign growth does not metastasize; a malignant one does. A benign growth does not destroy normal cells in the vicinity of its growth; a malignant one does. The benign cell is basically self-supporting; the malignant cells is a parasite, living off the nutrients it steals from normal cells.

All cells of the human body have the ability to reproduce themselves. Some cells—for example, the cells of the skin, bone marrow, and blood—reproduce rapidly because they need to be replaced more often. Other cells—liver, for instance—reproduce very slowly.

The process by which a cell reproduces itself is called *mitosis.* Normally, as the cell divides, it produces an exact duplicate of itself. Sometimes, however, a *mutation* occurs. Something goes wrong in the duplication process; the gene that manages growth and reproduction is damaged in some way. The result is flawed cells that seem to be arrested in the cycle of division and reproduction. Most normal cells have long dormant periods. The malignant cell, however, seems to have but one purpose: to reproduce endlessly. Unless stopped by the body's own defense system or some kind of therapy, cancer cells never stop reproducing. They continue to proliferate until they destroy the body that hosted their wild growth. Thus, a cancer is born when one cell loses control over its own reproductive system, beginning an unbridled spiral of growth that eventually becomes a tumor invading the area around it and even beyond.

What Is a Breast Cancer?

Ordinarily the various cells of the breast are dormant for long periods, producing new cells occasionally, as needed, and primarily during pregnancy. But when a cell in the breast departs from its usual dormant behavior, it becomes locked into a never-ending cycle of division and growth.

Two different types of cancer cells may appear in the breast. One of these—very rare and attacking mostly younger women and adolescents—is a growth in the fibrous tissue of the breast and is called a *sarcoma.* Much more prevalent is the *carcinoma,* a malignant tumor that originates in the more specialized tissues of the breast, particularly the ducts and glands. Unlike the sarcoma, the carcinoma is more likely to be a disease of advancing age and is related to the aging process. The term carcinoma is used to cover more than fifteen different varieties of breast cancer. Some of these varieties are rapid in their growth, while others are very slow.

There are other cells which are borderline between benign and malignant. These are clusters of cells so small that they cannot be seen with the unaided eye. Called *dysplasia,* they are thought by some physicians to be harmless. Nevertheless, many surgeons, fearing that these will grow into true cancers, argue for the removal of the entire breast to eliminate that possibility. (As we were to learn from many sources: some surgeons will perform a mastectomy when there is no evidence of cancer, if they think there is some chance of a future cancer!) Other physicians strongly disagree with this practice, citing the fact that these same dysplasia are often seen in the thyroid gland—and, in the male, in the prostate—where their presence is not regarded as harmful or indicative of a need for surgery.

There is also another type of growth that is somewhere between benign and malignant: the *in situ growth. In situ* means *in place,* and it refers to growing cancer cells that have remained in the area of origin, walled off, in a sense, from the rest of the tissue, lacking the ability to invade the tissues around them. They are cancerous in the way that they multiply, but they are like benign cells in that they are noninvasive. The usual treatment for this type of growth is the surgical removal of the tumor alone. In the

United States and Europe between 5 and 10 percent of the breast carcinomas are of this type.

Breast cancers are differentiated according to the types of tissue attacked in the breast. There are five main types of tissue in the breast: (1) the milk-secreting gland cells, (2) duct cells that carry the milk from the glands to the nipple, (3) the fibers that form the framework of the breast, attaching it to the chestwall and supporting it, (4) the fat cells that cushion the breast, making it comfortable and graceful, and (5) the lymph cells that are part of the lymphatic system and therefore part of the body's immune system. If a cancer originates in the milk glands, it is called a *lobular carcinoma.* Approximately one-fourth of all breast cancers originate there. If a cancer originates in the duct cells, it is called an *intraductal carcinoma* and three-fourths of all malignant tumors in the breast are believed to begin in the ducts. Very few malignant growths originate in fibrous or fatty tissues or in the lymphoid cells. However, once a cancer has originated in a duct or gland cell, it may eventually reach out and affect these other tissues.

Essentially separate from the breast are the axillary lymph nodes. The lymph cells assist the breast as they do the rest of the body by carrying waste materials from the tissues and functioning in the immune system—the body's own self-defense system. The lymph nodes are part of the breast's line of defense against cancer, attacking cancer cells and often destroying them. At the same time, the cancer cells may either overwhelm the lymphocytes or slip by them "in disguise" and spread into remote parts of the body. Thus the lymph nodes are both a defense line against cancer and an avenue for its spread. Next to the blood vessels, the lymph nodes are the most direct avenue for the spread of breast cancer. That is why the treatment of the lymph nodes—either by surgery or radiation—is often so important in the treatment of breast cancer. In testing for cancer, therefore, we must determine not only whether the lump in the breast is benign or malignant, but whether, if it is malignant, the cancer has lodged in any of the axillary nodes as well. This is one of the reasons for the early popularity of the radical mastectomy: both breast and nodes are removed in order to reduce the danger of the cancer having spread from the breast to the nodes. This is a critical issue to which we will return in the next chapter.

Cancers of the breast are classified not only in terms of the tissues they attack, but also according to stages of growth. This process of classification, called *staging,* helps the physician to determine what therapy will be needed and how extensive it should be. These stages are also used to compute statistics on both the control of cancer in the breast and the life-span that may be statistically anticipated. Over the years different physicians have used various classifications and criteria, but today the following is the most widely used:

Why are these classifications important? There are two reasons.

First, the type of treatment is dependent upon the particular stage at which the breast cancer is diagnosed. When a cancer is in Stage I or II, it may be treated either by surgery (mastectomy) or lumpectomy with radiation* . When it has reached Stage III, however, there is a high probability of metastasis to another part or parts of the body. In this case, surgical removal of the breast cannot affect the course of cancer growth in other parts of the body beyond the breast and its nodes. Nevertheless, many

*Although in this book and elsewhere the choice is usually represented as being between surgery and radiation, the radiation therapy Valere experienced and advocated by most radiologists is actually a combination of surgery—a lumpectomy to remove the tumor—and radiation. The surgical difference is that while the mastectomy removes the entire breast, the lumpectomy removes only the lump. Radiation alone—without removal of the tumor—has not proved to be a satisfactory technique.

STAGE	SPECIFIC CLASSIFICATIONS			EXPLANATION*
Stage I	T1a	N0	M0	Cancerous growth limited to breast
	T1b	N0	M0	
Stage II	T0	N1b	M0	Cancerous growth in breast and/or nodes, but not spread beyond
	T2a	N0, N1a or N1b	M0	
	T2b	N0, N1a or N1b	M0	
Stage III	Any T3	N1 or N2	M0	Cancerous tumor larger with or without nodal involvement
Stage IV	T4	Any N	Any M	Cancer believed to have metastasized to other parts of body
	Any T	N3	Any M	
	Any T	Any N	M1	

CLASSIFICATION CODES

T0	No evidence of primary tumor	N1a	Nodes not considered to contain growth
T1	Tumor 2 cm or smaller	N1b	Nodes considered to contain growth
T2	Tumor between 2 and 5 cm	N2	Nodes contain growth and fixed to one another or other structures
T3	Tumor larger than 5 cm	N3	Nodes near clavicle contain growth
T4	Tumor of any size attached to chest wall or skin	M0	No known distant metastasis
a	Tumor not fixed to fascia and/or muscle	M1	Cancer has metastasized to other part(s) of the body
b	Tumor fixed to fascia and/or muscle		
N0	No nodal involvement		

*The chart above is a condensation of classification material in *Clinical Oncology for Medical Students and Physicians: A Multidisciplinary Approach,* The University of Rochester School of Medicine and Dentistry, published by the American Cancer Society, 5th edition, 1978.

surgeons will perform a radical mastectomy on Stage III cancer patients, to no purpose whatever.

Secondly, when comparing the statistics for survival between patients receiving only radiation and those undergoing the mastectomy, we will find that Stage I patients are more successfully treated, in general, than Stage II, and so on. Staging, therefore, gives us a relative idea of the statistical possibility for cure and prolongation of life.

How Fast Do Cancers Grow?

In attempting to answer this question, we must keep the following things in mind:

1. All cancers do not grow at the same rate. Breast cancers are comparatively slow-growing.
2. Different kinds of breast cancers grow at different rates. The slower-growing cancers are usually easier to treat successfully.
3. The rate of growth of a particular cancer of the breast may not remain constant, so that there may be periodic slowing down or speeding up.
4. Since a cell grows by "twinning" or "doubling" itself, it may take a relatively long time for a single cancer cell to grow large enough to detect. However, because it doubles in size each time it reproduces, it grows very rapidly as a tumor.

Therefore, a malignancy begins as a tiny cell unseen by the human eye and it grows like this:

$$1 + 1 = 2$$
$$2 + 2 = 4$$
$$4 + 4 = 8$$
$$8 + 8 = 16$$
$$16 + 16 = 32 \text{ etc.}$$

In other words, five reproductions (or doublings) make the cell 32 times its original size. Ten reproductions will produce a growth 1,024 times its original size. Twenty reproductions will produce a growth 1 million times the original size and the growth will weigh approximately one gram. One additional reproduction will double the size of the growth to 2 million cells and 2 grams—and now it is large enough to be felt in the breast. Ten more reproductions will create a tumor of more than *2 billion* cells and weighing several pounds! (1cc = 10^9 cells).

How long does it take a cancerous breast cell to double or reproduce? As we have previously indicated, breast cancer cells are relatively slow in growth, requiring 50 to 150 days for the doubling process to occur. Inasmuch as it takes approximately 20 reproductions or doublings to reach a size of 1 cm., the fastest-growing breast cancers take approximately 1,000 days or 3 years to reach a size that is *palpable* or capable of being felt in the breast by touch examination. Thus a tumor that is discovered by either the patient or an examining physician is at least three years old, although, it is believed, it could be as much as seventeen years old.

Before the tumor may be felt by hand, however, it may have sent out cancerous cells to other parts of the body. If these cells find a receptive environment, they may begin to grow at the same slow rate as the parent tumor in the breast. Thus, by the time a tumor is large enough to be detected and treated, another cancer may be growing slowly in another part of the body. That is why it is important to examine not only the breast and nodal tissues, but also to check other areas of the body where breast cancers can spread and grow, such as the bone marrow, the liver, the lungs, and so forth. If such a distant cancer is discovered by a procedure such as a bone scan or liver scan then in addition to treating the cancerous growth in the breast, it will be necessary to select a therapy for the treatment of the distant cancer as well. Removing the breast, therefore, may be comparable to locking the barn after the horse has gotten out.

Radiation and surgery are techniques for attacking cancer of the breast and surrounding nodal areas. They are moderately successful in checking the spread of cancer to other parts of the body only if the cancer has not already metastasized before the therapy is administered. They also are effective in preventing the occurrence of cancer in the same breast. The possibility of such a recurrence relates directly to the stage at which the original breast cancer is detected.

How Do I Know If I Have Breast Cancer?

Most breast cancers are discovered by the patients themselves, rather than by their physicians. Valere, as well as many other patients to whom we've spoken, found her lump shortly after her routine examination by her OB/GYN physician. When a lump has been discovered (or some discomfort that suggests a possible lump) and the patient brings it to the attention of a physician, he may examine her himself or, as in Valere's case, he may send her directly for a mammogram—an X-ray picture of the breast. (Sometimes a patient will be given *thermography*, a technology that searches for tumors by means of heat detection. This technique, currently being improved and refined, is still too inaccurate to replace mammography.)

When a mammogram indicates the likelihood of cancer or at least a questionable area, a biopsy will be prescribed for the patient. These are the options then available:

a. If the character of the lump and the mammogram report suggest that the lump may be a cyst, the biopsy may be performed in the doctor's office with a needle and syringe. This is called *aspiration* and the fluid removed is examined by a pathologist to determine if any cancer cells are present.
b. If, instead of being filled with fluid, the lump is solid, a needle biopsy—taking out a sample of tis-

sue—may be performed in the doctor's office. Because this procedure requires a specially trained pathologist for diagnosis, it is not often available to the patient as an alternative procedure in many communities.

c. If, instead of a cyst, the suspicious area is discovered to harbor a tumor, the entire lump will need to be removed. This may be done in either a doctor's office or in the hospital. The removal of the entire tumor is the more likely procedure in most cases.

When breast tissue is removed in a biopsy, two laboratory tests are usually performed. The first is called a *frozen section,* a quick method that requires only fifteen to twenty minutes for a diagnosis. A small portion of tissue is cut and sent to the laboratory, where it is frozen and stained so that the structure of the tissue can be examined under a microscope. While the patient is still under anesthesia in the operating room, the surgeon awaits the diagnosis of the pathologist. In the past—and still all too often in the present—a frozen section biopsy interpreted as indicating malignancy was usually sufficient to motivate the surgeon to perform a radical mastectomy immediately.

Although the frozen section is stoutly defended by many surgeons today, it is a controversial procedure frequently attacked as lacking consistent accuracy. The freezing technique itself tends to distort the cells and the tissue may be distorted by the process of cutting, freezing, and staining.

Considerably more accurate is the second test, known as *permanent section.* This test is performed even if there has been a frozen section. It is a much more careful and painstaking procedure that provides a better picture of the cells and tissues under examination. The permanent section biopsy laboratory report requires three to four days before a diagnosis can be rendered. Although the permanent section laboratory report usually confirms the diagnosis of the frozen section, sometimes—and even once would be too often—the permanent section report does not agree with the diagnosis based on the frozen section. In short, some tumors pronounced malignant by the frozen section are discovered to have been benign. This means that from time to time a breast is removed on the strength of the frozen section diagnosis, which later is proved to be inaccurate or inadequate. If this is the case, you may be sure that the patient is *not* informed that her mastectomy was in error. None of the women we have interviewed were ever given that information.

Another advantage of the permanent section over the frozen section is the opportunity—at least in major medical centers—to do the test on an outpatient basis. The patient, after a few hours in the hospital under a local anesthesia, can go home the same day while the pathologist takes the necessary three to four days to return a complete report. The permanent section also permits a woman to request a second opinion from a pathologist at another medical center. This is not possible with the frozen section.

Too many mastectomies are still being performed on the basis of the frozen section. The time has come for women to demand the best diagnosis available from the biopsy.

Why Not Get It Over With?

If Valere had followed the advice of Dr. Moses, her entire breast and some nodes would have been removed on the strength of a frozen section. Had the permanent section laboratory report later indicated that the tissue was not cancerous, it would have been too late to change our minds—although we probably never would have learned of the error.

From our conversations with breast cancer patients, interviews with physicians, and from articles in the news media, we must conclude that large numbers of American women are still being rushed to mastectomy surgery on the basis of this one-step procedure: while the patient is still on the operating table, a mastectomy is performed on the basis of the frozen section biopsy without waiting the necessary several days for the permanent section laboratory report. There is no opportunity to confirm the frozen section biopsy as accurate, nor is there opportunity for the other highly necessary tests, including X rays, blood tests, liver scans, bone scans, and so forth. All this should be known *before* the woman makes her choice either for mastectomy or lumpectomy with irradiation. Furthermore, if the woman chooses a mastectomy, she needs to have ample time to choose among the surgical alternatives: radical, modified radical, extended radical, simple, and so forth. The surgeon's compulsion to get it over with robs her of both her right to know and to choose.

Dr. Luther Brady believes that between 80 and 90 percent of all women in the United States who submit to the radical or modified radical mastectomy are subjected to the mastectomy without benefit of the permanent section laboratory diagnosis—in other words: on the basis of the frozen section. However, Dr. Brady acknowledges that some of these mastectomies may be partly based upon other tests—for example, a needle aspiration—in addition to the frozen section.

In 1979 the National Cancer Institute strongly recommended that physicians use the two-step procedure, delaying decisions on modes of treatment until after the permanent section report as well as other testing procedures. Evidence indicates that the patient loses nothing if there is a reasonable interval *after* the biopsy in which she can consider alternatives.

An article in the *Dallas Morning News* in May, 1980, claimed that pathologists in that city believe a majority of women undergoing breast cancer surgery still are offered nothing but a one-step procedure, despite the recommendations of the National Cancer Institute. One prominent

Dallas breast surgeon was quoted as rationalizing his continued preference for the one-step procedure on the grounds that it saves time, expense, and mental anguish (although no breasts!). "If they want to spend the extra time and money in the hospital, we will do them that way too," he conceded.

Another local physician, however, disagrees. Dr. William Fry, chairman of the University of Texas Southwestern Medical School surgery department, believes that the two-step method not only has psychological benefits for the patient, but believes that when the biopsy is done on an outpatient basis, it can be more economical.

A more recent (August, 1981) check with a number of Dallas physicians indicates that Dr. Fry is not alone in his advocacy of the two-step procedure. Dr. Dale Fuller, a Dallas radiotherapist affliated with St. Paul's Hospital, told us that largely because of the information on this subject in the lay press, more physicians are coming to realize that the two-step procedure is important to both patient and physician.

Even if the two-step method were proven to be expensive—which it has not—it appears that this method is far superior from the point of view of patient morale, as well as in the interests of individual choice of therapy. In his presidential address to the American Radium Society in Las Vegas in 1977, Dr. Luther Brady underlined the medical advantages of the two-step procedure:

> Appropriate workup of the patient with cancer of the breast includes chest films, biochemical profile, complete blood count, and radionuclide liver and bone scans, all done within the context of a careful, complete history and physical examination. It seems appropriate to recommend that lumpectomy be carried out, the diagnosis of cancer established, and a metastatic workup performed prior to the choice of treatment. Unfortunately this is not done with regularity.

Data accumulated by the National Cancer Institute breast cancer epidemiologic studies indicate that most patients do not have appropriate workup prior to the selection of treatment.

Thus, the evidence is strong in favor of separating the biopsy from possible surgery or irradiation with an interval so that the patient can be adequately informed and be able to make her own choice. This is not a new idea. It is, in fact, standard procedure for many types of cancer other than breast cancer: first the biopsy and the diagnosis, followed by tests to determine if cancer has spread to other parts of the body. Only then is the decision made for a specific therapy plan.

Why, then, have surgeons traditionally rushed their breast cancer patients into surgery before all the facts are in? A possible answer is that it was formerly considered dangerous to delay the full amputation of a cancerous breast once any degree of surgery had been performed. There is no longer any reason to continue in this line of reasoning—and surgeons know it.

In addition, in earlier days, physicians did not realize how diverse breast cancers may be. In 1979, according to a report of the American College of Surgeons' Commission on Cancer, fourteen different kinds of breast cancer were discovered in examining 23,777 tumors. Some of these cancers were types that are slow in growth, some that are fast growing and spread quickly. All of this indicates that different strategies are needed in dealing with different kinds of cancers. None of these distinctions, however, can be made when the one-step frozen section method is used; it cannot provide that kind of information.

Even if the patient decides that she will choose some form of mastectomy, the one-step procedure is still inadequate. The National Cancer Institute has recently recommended that radical mastectomies not be performed on women with Stage I and Stage II breast cancers. But a truly informed diagnosis of the cancerous growth cannot be determined with the frozen section alone. Without the two-step procedure, the decision for a radical or a less-than-radical mastectomy is left solely in the hands of the surgeon—and on the basis of incomplete information. And it would seem that many surgeons choose to ignore both the National Cancer Institute's request on radical mastectomy and its plea for the two-step procedure. At a meeting of the American Cancer Society in September, 1979, when approximately 800 physicians were asked whether they use the one-step or two-step routinely, the show of hands indicated that only 50 percent had opted for the two-step. Thus, of the approximately 111,000 American women who will learn each year that they have breast cancer, one-half of them—55,500—will have to face the difficult task of choosing their therapy without adequate information about the various choices available to them.

The woman whose breast mammogram has suggested the possibility of cancer is not likely to learn from her physician that: (1) she may have a two-step procedure and (2) that, she will have several therapies from which to choose if the laboratory report indicates cancer. If she asks about the alternatives, she may incur the wrath of her physician, if not his out-and-out refusal to operate later on. One Dallas breast surgeon says that many surgeons he knows won't even discuss lumpectomy with their patients. "They refuse to discuss the procedure and refuse to refer them to doctors doing the procedure," he said. "They tell them just to go someplace else."

In the summer of 1979 a group of women went to Springfield, Massachusetts, to complain to the state legislature that they were unable to get necessary information about breast cancer. The group met with state Senator Carol Amick and told her that doctors were uncooperative in providing information beyond the mastectomy. One woman was told that without the mastectomy, she would die. Another woman consulted five doctors before she learned about the Joint Center for Radiation Therapy at Harvard.

The women wanted a law to protect the public's right to know and Senator Amick agreed. She recalled that there were far too many hysterectomies a decade ago, until public attention was drawn to them. The Senator encouraged the women to testify before the Massachusetts Senate Committee on Health Care. As a result a patient's rights' bill was enlarged to contain the specification that patients have the right to "complete information on all alternative treatments which are medically viable." Failure to comply with this legislation puts the physician in jeopardy of losing his license.*

Although legislation of this sort may appear to be an extreme measure, perhaps nothing less will suffice. In our own experience, neither of the surgeons we consulted presented radiation as a viable alternative. They did not say, "Here are two approaches, but I believe the mastectomy is the best." What they said was that the mastectomy was the *only* choice for a reasonable and responsible person.

Nor did we find the American Cancer Society helpful. The pamphlets they sent to us trumpeted the need for early detection, self-examination, the availability of the Reach To Recovery rehabilitation programs for postmastectomy patients, and little else. None of the three pamphlets—"Answering Your Questions About Cancer" (1977), "Breast Cancer Is Curable" by Phillip Strax (1974), and "Cancer of the Breast" (1975)—suggested that there was a choice between radiation and surgery. Chemotherapy was not even mentioned. In the second pamphlet, Dr. Strax declared that although the best treatment must be determined for each individual case, "at this time, surgery is the most effective treatment of breast cancer." Period.

---

*A similar law is now in effect in California.

Not a word about radiation. No mention of the two-step procedure as an alternative.

Actually, the most specific communication from the American Cancer Society was Dr. Jowl's Xerox copy of the circular letter (June 20, 1973). Indicating that the removal of the whole breast is the only viable procedure, the paper goes on to say:

> Recently, publicity has been sought about the possibility of not removing the breast and using limited procedures instead, with or without postoperative radiation therapy, for some cases of breast cancer. The basis for recommending limited surgery rests upon reports of only a few studies, particularly those done outside the United States, which suggest that survival from breast cancer discovered *early* and treated by limited surgery plus radiotherapy is equal to the results of removal of the entire breast. However minimal surgery must be consistent with prolonged survival, freedom from recurrence, and a satisfactory cosmetic and functional result.

Noting that studies are currently underway and that it will be years before the results can be made available, the paper goes on to indicate that "removal of the entire breast (most often the radical or modified radical mastectomy) is recommended for the surgical treatment of operable breast cancer. . . . Limited surgical procedures which remove less than the entire breast have not been sufficiently proven to be as effective as mastectomy."

In light of the statistics that were available when this paper was written, this is a remarkable statement. To write of radiation as "not sufficiently proven" without explaining that there is a considerable controversy within the medical profession on this matter, we believe, is irresponsible and removes the American Cancer Society from the position of an objective, scientific advisor to the American woman.

Immediately after Valere had finished her seed implants in December, 1977, I wrote the American Cancer Society, informing them that we were planning to write on breast cancer, and asked whether their 1973 policy statement was still in force. The reply from Dr. Arthur I. Holleb, senior vice president for medical affairs, assured me that "There has been no modification of the American Cancer Society's Policy Statement on the Surgical Treatment of Cancer since 1973. . . . Please do not interpret the statement as a 'warning' against the use of radiation therapy in the management of breast cancer. The sentence you may be misconstruing refers to limited surgical procedures with or without radiation therapy. The emphasis is on the surgical approach, not the adjunctive use of radiation therapy." If this is true—that the paper does not intend to warn against radiation therapy for breast cancer—then we must conclude that neither does it intend to acknowledge it as an alternative.

"Only preliminary results are available," writes Dr. Holleb, "and it will take many years before we can evaluate this technique in relation to standard forms of therapy." In light of the ream of medical papers on breast irradiation which I already had in my possession—papers to which I must assume he had at least equal access—I find it difficult to understand his ommissions.

He did worry that I, a mere layperson, should presume to write on breast cancer and wrote: "I trust you will not oversimplify a most complex and serious cancer problem which often requires individualization of management by a responsible physician". Finally, Dr. Holleb suggested that I contact a particular Dallas physician, "an expert oncologist who can answer all questions about breast cancer. However, he is an extremely busy man and may or may not be able to give you an appointment."

I already knew how busy this oncologist was and how unlikely it would be for him to further enlighten me. Dr. Moses had already told me what he thought of breast irradiation—and the people who chose it!

In a book which Dr. Holleb co-authored that same year with Jane Brody of the *New York Times, You Can Fight Cancer and Win,* Dr. Holleb cites once again what he calls "incomplete evidence" that lumpectomy and radiation are as effective in treating breast cancer as surgery alone. The evidence, in fact, he says, strongly "suggests that in the long run, radical surgery may save more lives." The question, then, he continues, "for women facing possible breast cancer surgery boils down to this: Is preserving both your breasts more important than maximizing your chances of living a full and healthy life?"

Nowhere in his book does he suggest that the woman ought to have the right to be fully informed about alternatives, nor that there is any value in a two-step rather than one-step procedure. He seems to regard the two-step method as a concession to the oversensitivity of some women:

> For women who insist on knowing the results of the biopsy before consenting to a mastectomy, surgeons have found that the chance for cure is not reduced if the operation is done as a two-step procedure—first the biopsy, and then a separate operation for the mastectomy should it be necessary. However, most women prefer to have the matter all taken care of at once rather than face two trips to the operating room.

The tone suggests that the reticence of the few is a manifestation of an inordinate concern for the preservation of the breast. Betty Leavell, one of the Dallas women who helped us to decide for irradiation, told us that her doctor said to her: "I can't understand why you are so concerned to keep both breasts. Why, I've lived all my life without breasts and it hasn't bothered me."

"Doctor," she replied, "if that were your penis we were considering cutting off, do you think you'd be so gung-ho with the scalpel?"

6.
If You Choose Mastectomy

TRUE or FALSE? Women who are closest to the medical profession—nurses, hospital employees, doctors' receptionists, members of a physician's family—because they know the value of early detection of breast cancer are more likely than others to seek early examination of suspicious lumps in the breast.

If your answer to this question was *true*, you are wrong. According to a surgeon who has specialized in the treatment of breast cancer, Dr. George Crile, Jr., emeritus consultant in surgery at the Cleveland Clinic, 25 percent of the women he and his colleagues treat for cancer of the breast that has become incurable because the patients neglected to seek early examination and treatment are "women who worked in hospitals, as doctors' receptionists, or who are members of a physician's family."

This is an amazing statistic—at least until you consider Dr. Crile's own interpretation:

> These women do not avoid treatment through ignorance of the diagnosis. They suspect they have cancer, but they have seen the results of radical operations. They defer treatment because they are more afraid of the mutilation than of the disease.

Thus it appears that with the exception of surgeons—few of whom are women—those closest to the medical scene and with an exposure to medical knowledge not in the possession of the general public are *more* afraid of the mastectomy, not *less*.

There is widespread fear of the mastectomy. According to Dr. Edward C. Saltzenstein and his associates at Mt. Sinai Medical Center and Medical College in Milwaukee, Wisconsin, many women refuse medical examination because of their intense fear of being hospitalized for a biopsy and waking up to find that one or both breasts have been removed. Obviously, and understandably, the loss of the breast haunts many women and often the men with whom they are intimate.

The surgical operation for the removal of the breast is known most widely as the *radical mastectomy*, or the *Halsted radical mastectomy*. For many people, the very name Halsted provokes fear and anxiety.

There is a certain irony in this. One hundred years ago when Dr. William S. Halsted, professor of surgery at Johns Hopkins, first pioneered the surgical operation that today bears his name, it was regarded with derision as a vain attempt to cure a disease that was regarded as incurable. Two prominent physicians, Dr. Samuel D. Gross and Dr. David H. Agnew, held that there was no hope for patients with breast cancer, and the great majority of physicians scoffed at Halsted's work.

Physicians advised their patients against the Halsted radical mastectomy. It was new—which was enough to damn it with some—and untried. There was no proof that Halsted could cure cancer of the breast with this preposterous procedure. Breast surgery had been attempted throughout the world with results that were universally disastrous.

That was in 1894. By that time Halsted had performed his radical mastectomy on just fifty women. The results were not startling—partly because of the seriously advanced nature of the cases that came to him—but he was convinced he was on the right track and he continued to perfect and refine his procedure.

It began to gain in popularity. Although the survival results were not outstanding and there were no studies available at that time on long-term data, other physicians began to join Halsted in using this procedure, and in a relatively brief period the Halsted radical mastectomy became *the* orthodox method of treating breast cancer.

Today the Halsted radical mastectomy is still the orthodox treatment for breast cancer. Almost a century has passed since this operation was introduced and it is essentially the same operation that Halsted performed. Although Halsted himself made some refinements of his techniques, in the last fifty years this operation has undergone no significant refinement or improvement. Nor has the survival rate for mastectomy patients improved during the last half century. The same percentage of women treated with the mastectomy are surviving or dying as indicated by statistics forty years ago. And, as Rose Kushner has pointed out in her book *Why Me?*, "The over-all survival rates of radical mastectomy are far from spectacular: a fifty-fifty chance of living longer than ten years after surgery."

How do radical mastectomies differ from modified radical mastectomies, simple mastectomies, and lumpectomies. What do these other terms mean, and how do they fit into the picture? Let's take a look at the different surgical procedures:

·*Radical mastectomy (Halsted)*—Removal of the whole breast, plus the fatty tissue surrounding it, the supporting muscles on the front of the chest, and all fat and lymph nodes in the armpit.

·*Modified radical mastectomy*—Removal of the whole breast and lymph nodes in the armpit. Usually, no chest wall muscles are removed, although sometimes some or all of the muscles may be removed and/or some of the lymph nodes in the armpit may be retained.

· *Simple mastectomy* or *total mastectomy*—Removal of the whole breast. Muscles and lymph nodes are left intact.

· *Subcutaneous mastectomy* or *mammoplasty*—Removal of all of the breast tissue, but nipple and skin are left intact so that in a later operation a silicone implant may be placed inside the skin.

· *Partial mastectomy*—Only a portion of the breast is removed and no nodes or muscles. The term *quadrant mastectomy* refers to the removal of one quadrant. *Wedge resection* or *segmental resection* refer to the removal of a segment of the breast. *Hemimastectomy* means the removal of one half of the breast.

· *Lumpectomy* (sometimes called *limited mastectomy* or *tylectomy*)—Removal of the tumor plus a small amount of tissue around it. (This is usually followed by radiation therapy.)

It is important to note that with the exception of the partial and limited mastectomy (terms rarely used or referred to), all mastectomy means the removal of the *whole* breast. The terms *simple* and *modified* lead some people to think that they are surgical procedures in which only a portion of the breast is amputated. These procedures differ, however, not in the amount of breast that is removed, but in the removal or retention of lymph nodes and muscle. Generally speaking, we may assume that the more radical the mastectomy, the more mutilation, discomfort, and impairment are likely to accompany it.

At one time, according to Dr. Ernest V. deMoss, a breast surgeon at the National Cancer Institute, surgeons assumed that "the bigger the operation, the more likely the cure." Today, however, says deMoss, "the current trend is to ask, 'What is the minimum amount of treatment that will give the same outome?' " The conclusion to which many physicians have come, says Dr. Joseph

Allegra, also of the National Cancer Institute, is that the radical mastectomy is no longer the preferred operation in breast cancers that are primary and localized and even those that have spread to the underarm lymph nodes. A nationwide study of 1,700 women, says Dr. Allegra, showed no difference in the long-term survival rates of women who had the modified radical versus the radical mastectomy. Dr. Allegra believes that breast surgery will gradually move to the simple mastectomy as the standard treatment until no one has a radical. An MIT researcher, Professor Maurice S. Fox, says that tests in Denmark and Great Britain also indicate that there is no survival benefit provided by radical mastectomy that is not equally provided by simple mastectomy plus radiation therapy. Similar results were obtained in the United States by the National Surgical Adjuvant Breast Research Study involving thirty medical institutions.

Yet despite these findings and recommendations by the National Cancer Institute,* many surgeons do not agree. Dr. Benjamin Byrd, chairman of the American Cancer Society Task Force for Breast Cancer Control and clinical professor of surgery at Vanderbilt University and Meharry Medical College in Nashville, Tennessee, told us (August, 1981) that he still believes that the "best proven method in treating invasive carcinoma involves the removal of the total breast and lymph nodes involved, because it is necessary to evaluate lymph node samplings." Dr. Byrd says that most of his breast operations are of the modified radical type. He performs the radical mastectomy only in selected cases.

It is difficult at this time to determine just how extensively this controversy has affected the practice of breast surgery in the United States. Some experts estimate that

---

*The National Cancer Institute has recommended against radical mastectomy for Stage I and Stage II breast cancers.

50 percent of the mastectomies performed in this country are the radical operation. Others have said as few as one in six. In *Choices: Realistic Alternatives in Cancer Treatment,* Marion Morra and Eva Potts maintain that the radical mastectomy is "the operation that most women in the United States with breast cancer routinely receive." The particular recommendation of the surgeon seems to depend on the age of the patient, her general health, size of the lesion, size of the breast, and the stage of the disease.

If you choose the mastectomy, what can you expect?

First of all, any mastectomy is major surgery. Even a simple mastectomy is not a simple operation. At the same time, it is not a dangerous operation. Normally people do not die from a mastectomy and it can be regarded as a very safe operation. A radical mastectomy may take from two to four hours compared to lumpectomies which require fifteen to thirty minutes. Your hospital stay will range from eight to ten days. Wounds from the more radical breast surgeries (radical and modified radical) will require from four to six weeks for healing.

When you awake from the anesthesia you may expect to experience some pain in the area of surgery. Usually a mastectomy incision is bound with a very tight surgical dressing to prevent the collection of fluid, which prolongs the healing process, and to reduce pain from coughing and turning.

For the first few days there will probably be some drainage tubes in the wound to carry away fluid and reduce swelling and pain. The chest and arm on the side of the surgery are likely to feel numb. This may go away in several weeks or months, but in a few people it remains as a permanent condition.

Of course, there will be a permanent scar at the site of the surgery; the more extensive the surgery, the more extensive the scarring. A radical mastectomy leaves a permanent hollow in the chest where muscle has been removed. As Kushner puts it, "I know of no clever ingenious ways to camouflage the scars left by that operation except sleeves and high necklines." When scars are extensive, skin grafts may be used.

Pain may subside in several weeks or last several months. In the case of a radical mastectomy, there is likely to be some permanent muscle weakness. In most cases there will also be some limitation in shoulder and arm movement, temporary or permanent. Regardless of the permanent or temporary status of pain or limitation, the arm should never again be used to take blood pressure readings, inoculations, vaccinations, or injections. Some physicians even warn against manicures and underarm shaving on that side. *Milk arm* or *lymphadema,* a swelling of the arm on the side of the surgery, is experienced by some patients on either a temporary or permanent basis, the latter requiring the permanent use of a postmastectomy sleeve which is similar to a support stocking worn for varicose veins.

When your mastectomy scar has healed, it is recommended that you be fitted for a prosthesis, a flesh-colored form that matches in size and shape the breast that has been removed. It may be inflatable, or solid, made from foam rubber or polyester and filled with silicone-gel, liquid, or air. A prosthesis is important, not only for appearance, but also to maintain correct posture and balance. There are also other pads that can be purchased to fill in depressions left by surgery.

Your physician will prescribe various exercises for you, or he may refer you to a nurse or physical therapist for this purpose. The aim of these exercises is to strengthen weakened muscles, regain the mobility of your arm, and prevent swelling.

Your doctor may also arrange for you to be visited by someone from Reach to Recovery, a volunteer program sponsored by the American Cancer Society. Women who have been through the convalescence of a mastectomy help others through the initial period by providing information and moral support. If you choose the mastectomy route, your surgeon can put you in touch with Reach to Recovery.

The mastectomy patient may experience profound emotional trauma. Dr. Kay R. Jamison and Dr. Robert O. Pasnau, two UCLA psychiatrists, have stated that the emotional suffering caused by the loss of a breast far outweighs the physical pain. In a survey of forty-one of their patients, they found that one out of four had contemplated suicide. One woman in their study was quoted as saying, "My deep depression has destroyed my libido. I have no sex drive at all. I am angry, hostile, outraged, and emotionally hate men, although not intellectually." Dr. Oliver Cope also has noted that "Immediately following mastectomy, anger is prominent." "Why me?" most women will ask, and it is not so much a question as it is a complaint.

Another emotional reaction is depression and anxiety. Many women are plunged into depression by the sight of their own wound and their breastless chest. Some will mourn their lost breast as they would a person. They will find it hard not to wonder whether their mastectomy is the end of their disease or just the beginning. Emotions may range from panic to grief. Some patients may cry a great deal, while others will lose their appetite or find it difficult to sleep or concentrate. Communication with family and friends may be difficult, if not impossible.

Most women will naturally worry about their marriage or love relationship. As one woman put it in an article in *Woman's Day,* "I'm terrified that [my husband] will be turned off by it all—that he won't find me attractive anymore." "It seems so unfair to have to worry about that too," another patient commented. For the unmarried woman the anxiety may be even greater as she worries how her mastectomy will affect future prospects.

Although there have been few intensive studies in this area, preliminary findings by some psychiatrists and counsellors indicate that most men respond more positively than women expect. A Connecticut psychiatrist who has counseled many people on this subject, has estimated that only 5 to 10 percent of the couples he has seen face major problems following the mastectomy. Another 20 percent, he says, may have moderate difficulty. Psychiatrists told Rose Kushner that in those cases where a mastectomy has been followed soon after by divorce, "those marriages were on the skids long before." A sound marriage, they assured her, will not be destroyed by a mastectomy. However, this is comforting only if a wife is assured that she has a good marriage and a mastectomy patient cannot help but wonder if her marriage is as good as she thought it was.

As may be expected, even though many men handle this situation with understanding and love, there are some who do not. Nevertheless, it seems that the greatest problem is not with the man and his attitude, but with the patient and her assumptions. Even though her mate may attempt to reassure her that the loss of the breast will not harm their relationship in general or their sexual activity in particular, the woman may be besieged by lingering doubts and suspicions. Recently on a flight back to Dallas from New York, Valere and I became engaged in conversation with the woman next to us. She was puzzled when she saw me taking notes from an article on breast cancer. In the course of our conversation she revealed that ten years ago she had gone to a hospital for a surgical biopsy of one of her breasts. Although she is certain that her surgeon never stated that he might go farther than a biopsy, when she awoke in her hospital room, both breasts were gone. A malignancy had been found in one breast and the other was removed by the surgeon, "just to be on the safe side."

Despite her husband's assurances that his love for her was unaffected, the woman told us that she was obsessed with the suspicion that he didn't mean it or that in time he would turn to someone else for his sexual fulfillment. At her insistence, the marriage ended in divorce. Today in retrospect, she realizes that her obsessive fears and anxieties detroyed the relationship.

Another woman reports her own postoperative feelings in an article in *Good Housekeeping:*

> I saw myself now as only *part* of a woman. Not really old, but never young again, either. I was deeply ashamed of the way I looked.
> Yet my husband acted as if nothing at all had happened. While I was falling apart, piece by piece, he continued on as if everything was still the same. Maybe he was trying to help me, but the distance between us seemed to grow.

Other couples report satisfactory adjustments and even, in some cases, a deepened relationship and growth in the marriage. Counseling may be helpful to most couples, as well as the previously mentioned Reach For Recovery program and a similar one, Encore, sponsored by the YWCA.

Still, many researchers and physicians question, whether it is necessary, in many breast cancers, for women to go through the physical and emotional trauma of the mastectomy at all. For example, Dr. Oliver Cope has written of the mastectomy:

> Surgery came on the scene when there was no other treatment of note. It brought relief and hope. Still useful in a limited way, still needed to help establish the diagnosis, major surgery as therapy has had its day. Mastectomy in any of its forms is on its way out.

Why is the mastectomy not being refined and improved today? The answer is simple: there is nowhere for it to go. The procedure has progressed as far as it can. In most branches of medical science, techniques may not last even a decade before they are substantially changed or replaced. If there was any way to improve the mastectomy —radical or otherwise—you may be sure that the surgeons would be doing just that.

Dr. George Crile, Jr, whose father pioneered the modified radical mastectomy in 1900, has made a stinging judgment on the Halsted radical mastectomy: "The operation that . . . is widely known as Halsted's radical mastectomy seems to have been designed to inflict the maximal possible deformity, disfiguration, and disability."

I think Dr. Crile is somewhat unfair to Dr. Halsted. The problem it seems to me is not with Halsted's contribution to medical science, but with those of his disciples who have, as Crile puts it, "perpetuated it with dogmatic fervor." For in making Halsted's approach dogma, they have tended to obscure that that approach was partly predicated on what has been proven to be a false assumption. Halsted designed his surgical procedure in the belief that breast cancers always spread first to the muscles and the lymph nodes nearest the malignant breast. Thus the heavy emphasis on removing as much tissue near the breast cancer as possible.

We now know that cancer may spread throughout the body without affecting the tissues adjacent to it. A single malignant cell may travel through the bloodstream to remote parts of the body. Therefore, by the time even a minute tumor is treated either by radiation or mastectomy it may have already metastasized to another part of the body. Survival of breast cancer patients will depend largely on how far the cancer has spread before the beginning of the treatment.

Dr. Cope found this evidence "so convincing that I did my last radical mastectomy in 1960." But other surgeons will counter with the argument that the whole breast must be removed because of the multicentricity of many cancers. Pathologists, in examining tumors removed from the breast, often find microscopic potential cancers elsewhere in the breast. Surgeons maintain that these microscopic tumors might become true cancers in time. Others believe that these slow-growing cells are not ever likely to become true cancers or that the possibility is very slight.

Dr. Samuel Hellman, a radiologist at the Harvard Medical School, is one of the leading proponents of the radiological approach. In April, 1980, Valere appeared with him as the only lay member of a panel at a breast cancer forum at Hahnemann Hospital. During the panel discussion, Hellman said: "Few topics in medicine engender as much emotional response as the treatment of primary breast cancer. This is true of patient and doctor alike. The medical literature is charged with strongly worded statements for and against the necessity of mastectomy."

This has certainly been our experience. Too often the subject has been reduced to a good-guys-vs-bad-guys conflict. The emotions go so deep that some professionals behave in a most unprofessional manner. Men and women of science easily are transformed into men and women with an axe to grind (or a scalpel). Rebuttals are made, not on the basis of data, but on the level of a personal attack, such as the one leveled against Dr. George Crile, Jr., by a surgeon in the June, 1973, issue of *Esquire:*

> The trouble with Crile is that he advocates so many goddam different things. . . . He has introduced a sense of chaos into breast treatment. It's a free country, unfortunately. Too free. It would be very nice if we had some sort of Academy of Medicine like they do in Russia to set the rules. . . . All the stupid people blowing their mouths off and influencing other stupid people—that's why we have all these hijackings and everything else.

At the same time many surgeons, and others in the health field, have managed to keep their perspective and an open mind. Marcie Lynn, writing in *Parents Magazine,* tells of her fair and compassionate treatment by Dr. William Silen, surgeon-in-chief at Beth Israel Hospital in Boston, even though she chose to have a lumpectomy and radiation instead of the mastectomy he recommended. Instead of rushing her into surgery, Dr. Silen advised, "Don't rush. Best to take time to think things over and consider the alternatives." Having outlined the alternatives, Dr. Silen also called Dr. Robert Goodman, a Harvard Medical School radiation therapist, to arrange an interview for Marcie Lynn and her husband, so that they could make an informed decision.

Doctor Silen: May your tribe increase!

7.
If You Choose Radiation

"New and untried!"
"Proven ineffective!"
"Dangerous!"
"And it may maim you for life!"

These were the arguments our surgeon used to try to dissuade us from our decision to have a lumpectomy and radiation therapy instead of a mastectomy.

Other surgeons have echoed these arguments. Dr. Arthur Holleb and Jane E. Brody in *You Can Fight Cancer and Win* sum up the surgical party line with these words:

> The question, then, for women facing possible breast cancer surgery boils down to this: Is preserving both your breasts more important than maximizing your chances of living a full and healthy life? For women who have thought this question through carefully, discussing it with family members or close friends as well as their doctors, the overwhelming majority opt for the very best chance to live, a radical or modified mastectomy, over the alternative—keeping both breasts but possibly diminishing chances for survival.

The logic seems quite compelling unless we realize that most of the premises are, in reality, not based upon fact but upon opinion—and in some cases little more than sheer prejudice.

Let's take a look at these premises.

First of all, the use of radiation therapy as primary treatment for breast cancer is hardly "new." In 1901, approximately two decades after the introduction of the radical mastectomy by Dr. William Halsted in Baltimore, Maryland, a Chicago radiologist, Dr. William A. Pusey, used "prophylactic irradiation" on a forty-five-year-old woman who had been submitted to surgery for breast cancer. Whether or not this was the first use of radiation for breast cancer, it is at least one of the earliest and indicates that breast irradiation is hardly fresh off the drawing boards.

Nor is it "untried." Here is just a sampling of some of the published studies that are available in medical literature:*

• In 1937 Dr. Geoffrey Keynes of England reported on the use of radiation for the primary treatment of breast cancer, some cases extending back into the 1920s, with a ten-year survival rate equal to that of patients who were treated by mastectomy.

• In 1954 Dr. S. Mustakallio of University Hospital in Helsinki, Finland, reported five-year survival statistics for 127 Stage I and Stage II patients of 84 percent. Although his radiation dosage is now regarded as inadequate, up to twenty years after therapy he observed no difference in

*In some of these studies, particularly the earlier ones, the lumpectomy was not always employed. In some cases, radiation therapy followed either a needle biopsy or incisional biopsy (in which only a portion of the tumor is removed). Research by J. Spitalier and others, however, as reported in the *International Journal of Radiation Oncology Biol. Phys.* confirmed in 1977 that the use of lumpectomy with irradiation substantially improved the potential for successful treatment. Today, lumpectomy is almost always combined with irradiation.

survival rates vs. surgery.

· In 1967 Dr. M.V. Peters of Toronto, Canada, reporting on 124 Stage I and Stage II patients, indicated a five-year survival rate of 76 percent, results almost identical to those acheived with surgery patients in the same institution.

· In 1969 Dr. P.M. Rissanean of University Hospital in Helsinki, Finland, reporting on 415 Stage I and Stage II patients, found a five-year survival rate of 79 percent, comparable to statistics for mastectomy patients in the same hospital.

· In 1971 three doctors at St. Helier Hospital in London, England, observing 96 Stage I and Stage II patients found a five-year survival rate of 94 percent for Stage I patients and 71 percent for Stage II. Comparable statistics for mastectomy patients in the hospital were 80 percent and 71 percent respectively.

· In 1972 four British physicians reported on 370 patients with five-year survival rates of 80 percent for Stage I and 60 percent for Stage II, compared to 80 percent and 75 percent respectively for mastectomy patients.

· In 1976 Dr. M.V. Peters updated her work with a report on 145 patients, some data going back thirty years, indicating that the radiation patients fared slightly better than the mastectomy patients.

· In 1976 physicians of the Yale University School of Medicine, Harvard Medical School, Hahnemann Medical College, and Jefferson Medical College reported on 150 Stage I and Stage II patients, with a five-year survival rate of 91 percent for Stage I patients and 60 percent for Stage II, comparable to results obtained with mastectomy.

More and more studies are being made available, but the consensus of the studies we have is that in Stage I and Stage II breast cancer patients, the survival and local control rates from radiation are equal to and sometimes slightly better than those from mastectomy.

In an article in the *New York Times,* April, 1981, "Traditional Treatments Joined by Promising Weapons," Jane Brody has this to say: "Radiation is increasingly being used in place of disfiguring surgery to treat early, localized cancers. . . . Thus far, high-dose radiation appears to be as effective as mastectomy in treating early breast cancer. Further study is needed to be certain of the long-term results."

Opponents of breast radiation therapy counter maintain that the studies are too few in number, too brief in the period of time they cover, and too selective in terms of the kinds of patients who are chosen for the radiation programs. The statistics, they say, are insufficient to prove that radiation is as effective as these studies seem to indicate.

Radiologists are quick to agree on the need for additional studies covering a broad spectrum of patients, but they believe that sufficient data now exists to justify offering radiation as a comparable alternative to mastectomy. In one of his papers, Dr. Luther Brady invites all sides of the controversy to do more intensive studies:

> The authors of these studies have never represented them as constituting definite proof. A well-designed prospective randomized trial of various treatment alternatives is necessary where each procedure being used is performed under ideal conditions.

Yet if the opponents of breast radiation therapy have their way, it seems to us, we will never have sufficient data.

At the same time, some physicians believe that the statistics with regard to mastectomy might be questioned. In personal communication with the author, Dr. John T. Chaffey of Harvard Medical School has said:

> When the surgical results are discussed they are always the results of those few centers who carefully follow and very carefully treat their cases. They may represent the very best

> in surgical practice. It is not often that a patient can ask her own surgeon what his personal results are and get a definitive answer. There seems to be some evidence that there may be a very wide disparity between the best results as quoted and the results the average patient is likely to obtain.

Dr. Chaffey acknowledges that this criticism may apply equally to researchers engaged in radiation studies and "only emphasizes the importance of each center and group keeping track of their own patients and honestly evaluating their own results."

The rough sampling of data outlined earlier in this chapter also refutes the claim that breast radiation therapy has been "proven ineffective." Even in those few studies where the data were slightly more favorable to the mastectomy than breast irradiation, we learn that these were early studies based upon data arising out of the use of radiation dosages which have since been proven to be inadequate. Opponents of breast radiation therapy frequently cite the 1972 report of J.J.B. Atkins of Guys Hospital, London, and others, because the results of their studies indicated that while the survival rate for Stage I patients was about equal for radiation and mastectomy procedures, Stage II patients with the mastectomy survived longer. What the critics fail to acknowledge is that Atkins and his associates used 3500 rads delivered over three weeks, a dosage no longer regarded as adequate by radiologists. This might be comparable to reporting that the local track and field star took ten minutes to run the mile race, while failing to mention that he did so with one foot in a plaster cast!

Some surgeons indicated to us that studies on the effectiveness of radiation in treating breast cancer are presently too few in number and cover too brief a period of time. It is true that in sheer numbers of patients, the results of the mastectomy are much better documented. It is also true that those results have been accumulating for the past century. But there is far more data now available to the medical profession regarding the effectiveness of breast irradiation than there was for the mastectomy when it was adopted as the standard therapy. Reviewing statistics from various breast irradiation studies, Dr. Victor A. Marcial, chairman of the Department of Radiological Sciences at the University of Puerto Rico, recently prepared a collation of that material for members of the National Breast Cancer Task Force and concluded: "Available data support the conclusion that tucorectomy [lumpectomy] and definitive irradiation for T_1N_0 and limited T_2N_0 lesions [Stage I and II tumors] gives equal clinical results as radical mastectomy in terms of five, ten, twenty, and thirty years survival without evidence of cancer." (March, 1981) How much more data is "enough?"

Thus, when breast irradiation opponents charge that in the long run—beyond five or ten years—surgery gives the only maximum chance of survival, they are citing not facts but opinions.

What all this means to you, is that from the data that is currently available, breast radiation therapy with lumpectomy indicates as good or better results in both local control and survival for stage I and II patients. Dr Luther Brady says: "Much suggested evidence has been accumulated that primary radiation therapy is as effective as mastectomy in the management of early stage breast cancer. It is even conceivable that it is more effective."

Dr. John Chaffey agrees, adding that breast radiation therapy "may possibly turn out to be even more effective since at least in theory we can cover a broader area of nodal involvement than the surgeon is able to remove."

The charge that radiation therapy for breast cancer is "dangerous" is equally unsupported by significant data. In fact, it seems reasonable to argue that the dangers from mastectomy are greater than those from breast radiation. For one thing, we have not been able to discover any general long-range or permanent negative effects. Some have given voice to the suspicion that radiation therapy may cause additional cancerous growths. While this is acknowledged as possible by radiologists, there is no data to indicate that this is true. It is frequently pointed out that we worry about the dangers of X-ray radiology using a very small dosage—for example, a tenth of a rad in a mammogram—while radiologists subject cancer patients to dosages of 5,000 or 6,000 rads. Yet, as Dr. Eleanor Montague professor of radiotherapy at the M.B. Anderson Hospital and Tumor Institute in Houston points out, just because a higher radiation dose is used, doesn't mean there is a higher chance of cancer. "A smaller dose, given over a longer period of time, is more carcinogenic (likely to trigger a cancer growth)."

One study indicated that the possibility of radiation-induced secondary cancers was well below the probability of surgery-induced malignancies.

It has also been suspected that radiation therapy to the breast would significantly reduce the body's immunological system, which normally protects us from cancer and other diseases. Clinical and laboratory data do not substantiate that claim. Furthermore, there is considerable dispute and uncertainy as to the role the immune system plays. In fact, in two studies with animal tumors researchers found that radiation caused less suppression of the immune system than did the surgical removal of regional lymph nodes, a standard part of the radical mastectomy.

Short-term or temporary effects can be few and minor, particularly when compared to the obvious and inescapable effects of the mastectomy. Many patients complete their entire course of breast radiation treatment without experiencing any side effects. In one study it was reported that 95 percent of the patients so treated "had no more than moderate radiation effects within the breast."

Among the temporary effects which some patients do experience are these:

Loss of appetite

Feeling of fatigue

Nausea with occasional vomiting, an effect that can be controlled by medication

Skin sensitivity, often compared to a severe sunburn followed by peeling

Esophasitis, a minor discomfort in swallowing, sometimes accompanied by a mild cough.

In the five-week program of outpatient treatment, Valere experienced considerable fatigue, some discomfort in swallowing, some nausea, and only in the final ten days a deep "sunburn" effect. Her greatest source of discomfort, then and in the months that followed, is a result, not of the radiation therapy, but of the discontinuing of hormone pills: intense hot-flashes.

Most women with breasts of average size have reactions similar to what Valere experienced. Large, pendulous breasts are likely to have a moisture reaction with the burn; in this case, it takes a little longer for the burn to heal.

Many people anticipate that breast radiation therapy will cause extreme symptoms such as falling hair or the loss of all hair. In all the literature we have examined and among all the people we have questioned, there has been no suggestion of that kind of radical effect.

Finally, there is the charge that radiation therapy may "maim you for life!"—our surgeon's actual words. Valere has examined the breasts of a number of women who have received the breast radiation. In each case the appearance has been excellent. Nor have we found any indication of poor cosmetic results from the therapy. Dr. Brady had told us that there would possibly be some minor changes in the appearance of the breast, barely perceptible changes in the contour, as well as a slight thickening. In addition, he said, the coloration of the treated breast might be just a shade darker. In our experience we have found that if you look for these differences you may just be able to find them. A little bit of Texas suntan has seemed to even out the coloration, leaving only a sprinkling of deep pink freckles.

Actually, the only visible sign of what Valere went through is the scar from the surgical lumpectomy. Even this, in time, will lessen in visibility, we have been told. It is said that in cases where a larger tumor is irradiated or a greater dose of radiation is used, effects of the therapy will be more visible. Yet, this is still greatly preferable to a scarred chest wall that no longer holds a breast. The charge that women who opt for breast radiation may be "maimed for life" is bewildering, particularly when one considers that every mastectomy patient is maimed for life.

When a woman chooses between mastectomy or radiation, there is another factor that needs to be kept in mind: radiation therapy is constantly being improved and refined. Dr. John Chaffey says: "We feel we are still in the process of learning how to deliver the irradiation effectively, locally acheiving the most desirable cosmetic result possible and still getting a high incidence of local eradication of the tumor." This means that, while present radiation methodology brings results equal to or better than mastectomy, further developments may both increase survival and control results and reduce still further the side effects for the patient.

In the earlier days of radiation therapy, Cobalt-60 machines were used extensively. Today these are being replaced by the more effective and more sophisticated linear accelerators. The techniques for shielding body parts that are not to be irradiated have also been greatly improved and refined.

By contrast, the art and science of the mastectomy has apparently reached its peak. As Dr. Chaffey told us, *the surgical treatment of breast cancer has failed to show any improvement in survival over the past thirty years!* The only changes taking place in the surgical community with regard to the treatment of breast cancer have to do with the argument for a less radical mastectomy than that which has been the norm in the past—and even this is a matter of considerable dispute. Regardless, a mastectomy—whether simple, modified, or by any other name—is still a mastectomy and requires nothing less than the complete removal of the breast. We do not think that it is at all incautious to say that breast surgery has gone about as far as it can—perhaps, even, too far.

In light of the demonstrated effectiveness of breast irradiation, it seems obvious that the deciding factor for many people will be the opportunity to save the breast without sacrificing the probability of survival or remaining free from the cancer.

Dr. Chaffey has observed: "Surgeons tend to downplay the importance to a woman of retaining her breast." We have found this confirmed in both our own experience and the experiences of others. Some surgeons chide their patients for their vanity in wanting to retain their breast(s) if possible. To be sure, a woman's ego has got to be involved in the possible loss of her breast. Her own self-esteem as a woman can hardly help but be threatened. The breast is part of her sexual identity. That doesn't mean she cannot live without it—people can and have adjusted to all kinds of physical handicaps and impairments. At the same time, most women may have considerable difficulty in making a complete adjustment to the loss, and some never do. We have heard our fill of stories of broken marriages (often, ironically, initiated by the woman), mental breakdown, and even suicide. The point is, women *can* live without breasts, but it is ridiculous, if not barbarous, to ask them to do so when there is a reasonable medical alternative.

While some surgeons are insensitive, others are downright cruel in their cavalier dismissal of the importance of losing a breast. We cannot help but wonder whether surgeons would be that insensitive if the majority of them were not men, but women.

Until now, we have spoken only of the merits and demerits of the two alternatives—mastectomy and radiation—in patients with Stage I or II malignancies. What about the choice when the cancer is diagnosed at Stage III?

There really is not much controversy when the cancer has reached this stage. It is generally conceded that radiation is the "treatment of choice," and mastectomy, if it is performed at all, is usually a partial mastectomy and is reserved for those patients whose primary tumors do not disappear during radiotherapy or those patients whose tumors show reactivation after initial response to radiotherapy and are unresponsive to chemotherapy.

The five-year survival rate for Stage III patients treated by either mastectomy or radiation is roughly about 26 percent. The reason for this discouraging statistic, of course, is that Stage III cancers are quite advanced in the breast, likely to involve surrounding nodes and/or chest wall, and may have spread to distant portions of the body. Once the cancer has spread to other parts of the body, the treatment of the breast, whether by surgery or radiation, can only effect the progress of cancer on the breast, not the distant malignancies. Thus, the chance of survival is greatly lowered.

Some radiologists believe that increasing the radiation beam dosage to 7000 or 8000 rads may bring better results with the Stage III cancers. Of course, this is likely to mean a more severe reaction of the breast and poorer cosmetic results. One way of surmounting this obstacle, some believe, would be to use a beam dosage of 4000 rads and increase the dosage of the needle implant to 4000. The use of chemotherapy with radiation and limited surgery may also considerably improve results with Stage III cancers.

It is important to note that there are variations in the methodology of breast irradiation. Valere's program, the standard program at Hahnemann and other similar institutions, consisted of: (1) radiation beam outpatient treatments of 200 rads per day, five days per week for five weeks, totaling 5,000, and (2) removable seed implants of iridium-192 using 2,700 rads over a four-day, inpatient hospital stay

Some radiologists have used only the beam treatments. One doctor, we found, uses only the seed implants. Some doctors advise the use of a needle biopsy, while most seem to recommend a lumpectomy. Treatment will also vary somewhat depending upon the location of the tumor on the breast, as well as its relationship to the surrounding area.

From all that we have observed and read, however, it appears that the best and most consistent results—in terms of survival, local control statistics, and cosmetic effects—have been obtained when the tumor is surgically removed by lumpectomy and the breast is treated with both the radiation beam and the seed implants.

There are two additional advantages from the use of breast radiation. Once freed of the fear of mutilation by surgery and the loss of the breast or breasts, women are more likely to accept the the need for self-examination and for speedy medical help if something suspicious is detected. Many women who find a disturbing lump or experience discomfort in the breast try to ignore it in the hope that it will eventually go away. This delay may cost the woman the difference between a Stage I, II, or III cancer.

Furthermore, there is an intangible factor that may come into play when a patient elects radiation therapy: freed of the fear of losing a breast(s), most women will develop a more positive attitude toward both their illness and their treatment. Although we have not yet been able to measure precisely the difference a patient's outlook may make, many physicians believe that morale is a very important factor, perhaps even crucial. (We will explore this further in chapter nine.) Obviously, it is much easier to maintain a positive attitude with both breasts intact, than it is without one or both.

Let's take a look at the balance sheet:

MASTECTOMY	BREAST RADIATION
1. Good results for both local control and survival in Stage I and II cancers	1. Equal or better results
2. Statistical data compiled over a long period of time	2. Statistical data limited in time and scope, but growing
3. Loss of the breast(s)	3. Retention of the breast(s) with good cosmetic results
4. Severe psychological trauma over the loss of the breast(s) often occurs	4. Emotional trauma greatly reduced, if not eliminated
5. Marital or other relational strains often may become serious	5. Minimal strain on relationships
6. Physical impairment and discomfort in the arm, shoulder, chest area usually results, sometimes permanently	6. Physical effects of radiation usually temporary and mild
7. Hospitalization and home recuperation of several weeks	7. Outpatient treatment with brief hospitalization for seed implants (when used) and little home recuperation
8. Prosthesis (false breast) required	8. No prosthesis needed
9. Technique development is static, remaining largely unchanged	9. Technique is constantly being refined and improved
10. Fear of self-examination and medical follow-up induced.	10. Fear reduced and both early detection and medical care encouraged, while maximizing the powers of morale.

The bottom line, it seems to us, is this: *Available data indicates that your chances for curing your breast cancer and survival are as good as or better with radiation than with mastectomy—and the cosmetic and psychological result is infinitely better.*

Unless, of course, you accept the argument that more data is necessary. Only you can make that judgment.

8. Are There Other Choices of Treatment?

The breast cancer patient has a right to know about and choose between the various alternative medical therapies. So far, we have looked at two of these: mastectomy and irradiation.

But why stop there? Are there only these two, or are there others about which we need to know?

In fact, what about all these other cancer "cures" we hear and read so much about? Chemotherapy? Hormone therapy? Immunotherapy? Vitamin C therapy? Hyperthermia? Dietary therapy? And interferon—isn't that supposed to replace them all? Yes, and while we've got this can of worms open, what about Krebiozen, Laetrile, the Hoxsey treatment, the Burton serum, the lactobacillus therapy, and the Kelley clinics? We've also heard about a mind control technique used by Dr. O. Carl Simonton, not to mention the claims some people have made for spiritual healing.

As we consider each of these, as well as breast reconstruction, we need to realize that in treating breast cancer with any therapies, we have four basic goals: (1) to get rid of the cancer in the breast (referred to by doctors as *local control*) and the chest area immediately adjacent *(regional control),* (2) prevention of recurrence of the cancer in breast or chest, (3) prolongation of life, and (4) maintaining the best physical appearance and condition possible (called *cosmetic results*).

If there is a later recurrence of breast cancer, it may appear in the same breast (if it hasn't been removed), the opposite breast, the nodes and muscles adjacent (called *axillary*), or other parts or organs of the body. When the disease has spread to other parts of the body, we say it has metastasized and the resulting cancerous growth is often referred to as a *distant, remote,* or *occult* (meaning *hidden*) cancer.

People do not die from breast cancer in the breast or even the nodes. They die from breast cancer that has spread to other parts of the body and caused the failure of other organs. For example, if cells from a cancer in the breast enter the bloodstream and are carried to the liver, where they prosper and grow, the patient will have a breast cancer in the liver.

As we've already indicated, both surgeons and radiologists acknowledge that surgery or radiation therapy (or both together) can be effective only in treating the cancerous tumors in the breast and the adjacent area, as well as preventing the spread of the cancer to other parts of the body. But if, when the breast is treated by surgery or radiation, the cancer has already metastasized to some other area of the body, neither mastectomy nor breast irradiation can have any effect on this "new" cancer, referred to as a *secondary* cancer (as the breast cancer is a *primary* cancer). In this case, it is said that the cancer is *systemic,* no longer confined to the local or regional area, but dispersed out into the body's systems.

In Stage I and II cancers (see chapter five) the mastectomy and radiation therapies have proven fairly successful in local control, prevention of recurrence, and survival of the patient. For example, in a ten-year study of 293 breast cancer patients at Yale, Harvard, Jefferson, and

Hahnemann medical schools, 81 percent of the Stage I patients and 54 percent of the Stage II patients were still alive ten years following treatment with lumpectomy and radiation. Of the 293 patients, only 23, or 8 percent, had a recurrence of breast cancer on the breast or adjacent area. Of these 23 patients, 10 are now apparently free of breast cancer following further surgical treatment. "These results," says Dr. Leonard R. Prosnitz of Yale, who reported for the hospital group, "are entirely comparable to the great majority of surgical [mastectomy] studies."

In addition, statistics from the ten-year study reveal that 85 percent of the patients had a good or excellent cosmetic result and only 15.3 percent had any treatment complications, none of these fatal and mostly mild—results, of course, superior to those from mastectomy.

Most of those patients who did not survive the ten-year period died as the result of metastases which took place prior to the radiation therapy (although some died of causes quite unrelated to cancer). Most of the alternative therapies we will be looking at in this chapter are intended to deal with breast cancer that has metastasized. They are intended for the most part to be used in addition to, rather than in place of, radiation or mastectomy.

Chemotherapy

Chemotherapy is the treatment of cancer with chemicals or drugs. Unlike the mastectomy and radiation therapies, it is not intended to treat the primary or breast cancers, but those that have spread beyond the breast.

When there seems to be a possibility that the breast cancer has metastasized, chemotherapy is usually recommended to treat the distant cancer that the mastectomy and radiation cannot affect. Because chemotherapy is used as a follow-up to either mastectomy or radiation, it is called *adjuvant therapy*.

Chemotherapy is used in breast cancer when:

(1) Laboratory or surgical sampling indicate that the breast cancer has spread to one or more axillary lymph nodes
(2) Laboratory tests indicate that metastases may have taken place. (Among the factors indicating this possibility are the stage of the cancer, the location in the breast, the aggressive nature of the tumor, the receptivity of the tumor to estrogen and progesterone, plus indications of vascular—bloodstream—and lymphatic invasion.)
(3) Various tests or other evidence indicate that the cancer has already begun to grow elsewhere.

What does chemotherapy do?

Chemotherapy drugs are toxic or poisonous elements that are harmful to the body's healthy cells, but even more injurious to cancer cells. Entering the bloodstream, they are carried by the blood to wherever tumors may be growing in the body. Cancer cells are particularly susceptible to chemotherapy drugs because, unlike healthy cells, they are constantly in the process of growth and reproducing. Chemotherapy kills cancer cells. If the tumor is small and the drug kills many cancerous cells, it may eliminate the tumor. More often—particularly if the tumor is large—chemotherapy will kill enough cells to retard or halt its growth. Usually we can say the smaller the tumor, the earlier its stage of growth, the more successful the drug is likely to be in eliminating it.

Originally, chemotherapy was used mainly to treat patients with advanced cases of cancer. For this reason, many people today mistakenly assume that chemotherapy is a measure of last resort or an indication that the disease is too advanced for cure. More and more physicians are using chemotherapy in the early stages of cancer when there is some reason to believe that cancer has spread.

At the present time, chemotherapy produces cures in about 15 percent of the cases in which it is used (although that rate seems to be climbing). Otherwise, chemotherapy is intended to retard the growth of tumors, relieve pain, or permit the patient to live a longer, sometimes more comfortable life. Sometimes chemotherapy has no effect upon the growth of the cancer.

Chemotherapy is relatively new in the treatment of cancer. Only since the 1940s have drugs been effective in destroying and retarding cancer cells. In the 1960s and 1970s there has been a rapid growth in the development of new drugs and the skill of administering them. Chemotherapy is rarely used by itself as a primary therapy and is usually combined with other techniques.

There are a number of different types of chemotherapy drugs. Some attack and try to destroy the cancer cells themselves. Others inhibit the secretion of hormones upon which some breast cancers are dependent (estrogen, adrenal cortical hormones, prolactin, and so forth). To date, approximately fifty drugs have been identified as being lethal to cancer cells. Of these, about twenty have been used in the secondary treatment of breast cancer, eight of them being particularly effective.

Usually, two to five chemotherapy drugs will be used in combination and often in rotation, requiring that the chemotherapy process be spread out over a period of months. Different drugs will be used on the same patient in order to attack cancerous cells at different phases of their reproductive cycle. They are used in rotation to minimize the chances of the tumor becoming resistant to one particular drug. Periods of administration average three weeks in duration at a time, with a rest period of six weeks to allow the healthy cells to recover from the effects of the toxins.

All the drugs currently being used in chemotherapy are toxic. In fact, that is why they are effective. Because cancer cells are human cells gone berserk—and not foreign invaders—a drug which is likely to be toxic to cancer cells is also likely to be toxic to healthy human cells, although not to the same degree. This is why there are side effects to the use of chemotherapy, slight in some people and with some drugs, and severe with others. Different drugs have different side effects and some people are more sensitive to some than to others.

Among the various side effects are: bone-marrow depression (affecting production of blood cells), chronic lung problems, skin darkening, hair loss, breast enlargement, impotence, sterility, kidney damage, hearing problems, bloody urine, loss of appetite, mouth sores, skin rash, poor muscle co-ordination, nail loss or brittle nails, gastro-intenstinal problems, coughing, fever, peeling or tenderness of the skin, headaches, swelling and pain in joints, unusual taste sensations, heart problems, chills, nausea, constipation, numbness or tingling in hands or feet, fluid retention, high blood pressure, loss of potassium, increased risk of infection, diabetes, lowered blood calcium, uterine bleeding, feminization, masculinization, jaundice, flu-like symptoms, delayed blood-count depression, mental depression, tremors, lethargy, and drowsiness. Please note that this list is for all fifty drugs and each drug may have only two or three side-effect potentials. As we've already indicated, some people do not get any reaction or their reaction is minimal. Most of the side effects, including hair loss, are temporary; most effects last a few hours to a few days. Because of the harm to normal cells and tissues, it is usually unwise to administer chemotherapy and radiation simultaneously.

Chemotherapy is a growing technology. We may expect that new drugs will be effective on cancer cells that are now resistive to drugs. Perhaps drugs will be developed which will be much less toxic—if not completely harmless—to healthy cells. Additional discoveries may eliminate or offset the toxic effects on the human body itself.

Many physicians, Dr. Oliver Cope among them, have hailed chemotherapy as "our first new hope in twenty-five years." Others are deeply concerned about the limits of the use of chemotherapy. In advanced diseases the use of chemotherapy may simply be to buy time for the patient. If the side effects are serious, the question arises as to whether drugs ought to be administered only to prolong life. We need to be as concerned with quality of life as with quantity of time. This is a decision which the physician cannot make for us.

But the promise of chemotherapy is its potential to keep early-stage cancers from becoming advanced. In 1977 a group of Milanese physicians under the direction of Dr. Gianni Bonadonna conducted a pioneering study of the use of chemotherapy as an adjuvant treatment in breast cancer. The 381 patients all presented a high risk of having a metastasized cancer as one or more axillary lymph nodes were affected. Although survival rates were not affected by the program, the rate of recurrence in the breast or adjacent region was significantly better with the patients who received the drugs (3.3 percent vs. 13.3 percent).

Another important study was carried on in the United States of America by the National Cancer Institute's Breast Cancer Task Force under the direction of Dr. Bernard Fisher of Pittsburgh and reported in 1976. The initial study involved 196 patients who had had a mastectomy with at least four lymph nodes found to be cancerous. Ninety-nine of the patients were treated with a combination of drugs; 105 were given a placebo (pills that contained no drugs, although patients thought they did). The group using chemotherapy fared considerably better in the statistics for recurrence. Treatment was found to be considerably more advantageous to women who had not yet experienced menopause.

One celebrated chemotherapy report—expanded Bonadonna studies in Italy—has been found to be premature in its claims. First reported in the United States in the February 19, 1976, issue of the *New England Journal of Medicine*, the results of the trials of CMF, a combination chemotherapy, were hailed as a work of "monumental importance" and the data were celebrated as "nothing short of spectacular." As a result of this report, major shifts in treatment philosophy were made in this country, a change affecting thousands of cancer patients.

Now, five years later, critics claim that initial responses to these studies were hasty and unwarranted. The more these CMF studies have been examined, the more disappointing the conclusions. Furthermore, toxic side effects have been found to be a considerable risk, including greater incidence of leukemia and second cancers. One of the critiques by Dr. Seymour H. Levitt and Dr. Roger A. Potish also cites British studies indicating a higher incidence of serious psychiatric illness with patients using chemotherapy (66 percent for patients with chemotherapy alone, compared with 25 percent for patients with mastectomy alone.)

In summary, chemotherapy, although still in experimental and developmental stages, can be used as adjuvant therapy after mastectomy or radiation to fight and even cure metastasized breast cancer in its early stages, as well as to reduce the growth and consequences of more advanced disease in remote parts of the body. We may assume that there will be considerable advancement in chemotherapy in the years ahead.

Hormone Therapy

Actually, hormone therapy is a kind of chemotherapy, the chief difference being that while most chemotherapy drugs attack the cancerous cells in the body, hormonal drugs attempt to affect—or add to—the body's own production of hormones which have an effect upon the growth of cancerous cells. Like chemotherapy, hormone therapy is not an alternative to the mastectomy or radiation, but an adjuvant supplement, used most often in connection with chemotherapy. It is used most often with rather advanced cases of breast cancer.

At one time the same results now achieved with hormone therapy were sought with various kinds of surgery, primarily the removal of the ovaries, and sometimes the adrenal or pituitary glands, all of which secrete hormones which may affect the growth rate of cancer in the breast. These surgical operations are rarely used today.

Depending upon the kind of cancer, hormone therapy has been used either to stimulate or shut down the production of hormones. Most often male hormones (androgens) are used in the treatment of advanced cases of breast cancer in women. Today, however, most hormone therapy is aimed at suppressing estrogen, and an anti-estrogen drug, tamoxifen, is used to compete with the estrogen manufactured in the body. Hormone therapy does not usually involve side effects.

One of the most important findings in the laboratory analysis of a biopsied tumor is whether the cancer's growth is affected by hormones, chiefly estrogen, a female hormone manufactured in the human body and also present in birth control pills. This test is called an estrogen-receptor (ER) test. If the test is found to be positive, 60 percent of the women who use hormone therapy will benefit from it to some extent (in retarding growth, not as a cure). If the ER test is negative, then less than 10 percent of the women in this group will benefit. A positive ER is found in approximately 60 to 70 percent of women with tumors that have metastasized. The ER test is accurate in approximately 75 percent of the patients tested.

Hormone therapy is moderately effective in the control of advanced breast cancer, but except in special cases it is not an alternative primary therapy. In the future, it could become a more important treatment.

Immunotherapy

Immunotherapy is well established in many fields, but at present it is little more than a hope in the treatment of cancer. Immunotherapy is an attempt to fight a disease by stimulating the body's own immune system to destroy the invading disease, usually by using small amounts of bacteria or other microorganisms. Immunotherapy is well established in combating smallpox, diphtheria, yellow fever, and polio, to name just a few.

The immune system—a whole complex of mechanisms in the human body—is the body's own defense system against disease. Common allergies are an illustration of the immune system at work, constituting an overreaction of body's protective responses to irritants. When we read of an attempted organ transplant—such as a heart transplant—and are told that the attempt failed because the body rejected the alien organ, it is an example of the body's own defense system against invasion from without.

Many in the medical profession believe that the body is frequently attacked by cancer-producing agents, but when the immune system is working to capacity, it is usually able to defeat the invasion without our even being aware that a battle has taken place. Thus, scientists have attempted to find ways and means of stimulating the body's own immune system to fight cancerous growths.

This research has proceeded along two lines: (1) the development of an immune reaction against possible cancer viruses (just as the body develops defenses against other viruses and bacteria), and (2) the development of an immune reaction to fight cancers that are not caused by viruses. Although it is believed by many that a virus is instrumental in some kinds of cancer, attempts to isolate these viruses have failed to date. Although viruses have been found to cause spontaneous breast cancers in certain strains of mice, no such virus has as yet been found operative in human breast cancer.

Some research using a bacterial agent to provide immunity from malignant melanomas has been carried on at UCLA and in France, but this research is in its infancy. We can only hope that significant strides may be made along these lines.

The patient's own immune system is the focus of two additional concerns related to both mastectomy and the use of chemotherapy.

Dr. George Crile, Jr. has warned surgeons against the removal of lymph nodes in the performance of mastectomies on breast cancer patients. The lymph nodes are part of the body's immune system and Dr. Crile believes it is important to leave these intact, when possible, to assist the body in fighting the cancer. Although his warnings were initially ignored and are still in dispute, other physicians have joined in cautioning against unnecessary removal of lymph nodes, except for the purpose of nodal sampling to detect the extent of the cancer. A study by Dr. M. H. Edwards and others supports this view and indicates that when axillary nodes were not removed, in 75 percent of the cases studied there was a spontaneous regression of the nodal cancer.

Another area of concern is the effect of chemotherapy on the immune system. Among the healthy cells of the body that are hardest hit by drugs are the lymphocytes and white blood cells, both essential agents in the body's immune system. This is why patients undergoing chemotherapy are particularly vulnerable to bacterial and viral infections. Others worry about the harmful effect of radiation on the immune system.* When these therapies are used despite their possible harmful effects to the immune system, it is because the immune system is not sufficient to halt the growth of cancer, while the therapies are effective.

---

*Studies by Dr. C.A. Perez and also Dr. Gilbert H. Fletcher suggest that irradiation to the regional lymph nodes is far less suppressive of the immune system than removal by surgery.

Interferon

Although we are listing interferon separately, it is actually a kind of immunotherapy since interferon is a protein produced by the body's own cells in response to some stimulation, usually a virus. Interferon acts as a kind of messenger that alerts other cells to the invasion of an adjacent cell in which a virus or other invader has gained control. Thus warned by interferon, the neighboring cells produce an antiviral protein which prevents the invader from gaining a beachhead.

Medical science is cautiously excited about the development of interferon because, unlike chemotherapy, interferon does not attack cells, but stimulates the body's defenses to isolate invasions. Furthermore, interferon seems to be effective against both viral invasions and tumors thought to be caused by nonviral agents. Side effects are limited, it seems, to slight fever, fatigue, and a small decrease in the bone marrow's production of blood cells.

The usually conservative American Cancer Society is so interested in interferon that it invested an initial $2 million for the first round of tests in the United States. Results so far are fragmentary, but look promising. The problem now is to manufacture sufficient quantities for large-scale experimentation at a reasonable cost. The current experimentation project by the American Cancer Society is limited to seventy patients with advanced cancer.

Although interferon gives promise of significant breakthroughs, it has been prematurely and overly celebrated by the media. There are still tremendous obstacles to be overcome. "In terms of research," says University of Wisconsin cancer specialist Dr. Ernest Borden, "we're only about 2 percent of the way along toward widespread clinical application." Even if the research continues to prove hopeful and the obstacles are overcome, interferon at present will most likely be used as a supplement to, rather than a replacement for existing treatment.

Breast Reconstruction

This is not a therapy at all, but a cosmetic measure used to restore the semblance of a breast following a mastectomy. It is not used, or needed, following lumpectomy and breast irradiation. In order for a breast reconstruction to be feasible, the mastectomy must be performed so that a sufficient flap of breast skin is allowed to remain. After the mastectomy wound has thoroughly healed (three months at the minimum), a plastic surgeon will perform one or more operations to reconstruct the breast, using the original breast skin and a rubber envelope of silicone gel. Several operations may be needed to fill in the chest wall when the mastectomy has been radical. The reconstruction, which may cost between $1,500 and $5,000, may involve the reconstruction of a nipple, if desired, but this usually requires another operation. Although most patients are pleased with their reconstructed breast(s), plastic surgeons warn that women must not expect that the reconstructed breast will be cosmetically equal to the amputated breast.

Both the American Cancer Society and the National Cancer Institute recommend that patients prepare for breast reconstruction at the time of surgery. It is possible to perform breast reconstruction later, but it is necessary to assure that sufficient tissue remains for the reconstruction. If tissue is insufficient, the reconstruction may not be possible. The more radical the mastectomy, the more difficult the reconstruction. Although a few surgeons will undertake breast reconstruction at the time of the mastectomy, physicians with whom we have spoken think this is a questionable procedure for the following reasons: reconstruction should not be performed until the chest wall is disease free, a process requiring approximately one year; the chest wall should be allowed to heal first; after the area is healed it will be easier to determine the size of the prosthesis needed.

Hyperthermia

Hyperthermia involves the use of heat to kill cancer cells. Heat in one way or another has been used in cancer treatment for centuries, although scientific evidence of its efficacy has been lacking and inconclusive. Actually, hyperthermia is a kind of immunotherapy, for heat seems to stimulate the body's immune system. Further research is being carried on, but there is no conclusive evidence available at this time. Even if the potential of heat as a cancer treatment is fully developed in the future, it is likely to be an adjunctive therapy and not a primary alternative.

Vitamin C Therapy

Claims for the effectiveness of vitamin C in large dosages in the treatment of cancer appear in the media from time to time and Dr. Linus Pauling has strongly advocated its use. Despite claims made for it, there are no published scientific studies that prove it is effective in treating cancer. That doesn't mean it isn't, but rather that we do not have research evidence at this time. To this end, the National Cancer Institute has funded a study at the Mayo Clinic in Rochester, Minnesota, to determine if vitamin C either relieves symptoms of cancer or extends the lives of patients. The study involves patients who no longer are responding to other therapies. If vitamin C is effective, it is likely that it will be found to be helpful to the immune system. At most, it would be a supplemental therapy. With few exceptions, there seem to be no side effects from the use of the vitamin C in the dosages prescribed by Dr. Pauling.

At this point, maybe the best we can say is that it probably can't hurt, and it may well help.*

The "Outlaw" Therapies

We've lumped together a number of claimed therapies which are either presently illegal in all or most of the United States, or, at least, are being carried on outside the medical establishment. These include laetrile, Krebiozen, the Hoxsey herbal treatment, the Lactobacillus bacteria advocated by Florida milk producer J. Gordon Roberts, the Kelley clinic programs, the serum of Dr. (zoologist) Lawrence Burton of New York and the Bahamas. One estimate places the number of these outlaw therapies at fifty.

By designating these therapies as outlaw, we do not mean to imply that they have been proven to be ineffective. Some have, some have not, but neither is there sufficient hard research to demonstrate that their claims are valid.

Some of the claimed therapies may be intentionally fraudulent, while others may be honest attempts to find viable alternatives. We have known a number of people who—failing to find help in conventional medical therapies—have appeared to benefit from one or more of these. For example, a friend in Florida, given up as hopeless by medical science, was convinced that her survival many years beyond her medical prognosis was due entirely to her participation in the Kelley clinic (which utilizes vitamin supplements, dietary management, and coffee enemas), at that time located just outside Dallas. Whether there was value in this treatment or whether her remission was the result of other factors, including her own

*The research of Dr. Ewan Campbell of Scotland does indicate that vitamin C may prolong survival time of the cancer patient, even if it does not cure.

belief in the treatment, is impossible to determine. (More on the possible power of belief in chapter nine.)

One of the outlaw therapies which is at last receiving some attention from the medical establishment is Laetrile. Having long opposed the use of Laetrile without having done any research, the scientific community is at last responding to enormous pressures from the lay public with a series of tests. The National Cancer Institute conducted tests of Laetrile in 1957, 1960, 1969, 1973, and 1975, all using mice. They concluded from these tests that Laetrile was not proven to be effective in combating cancer. Supporters of Laetrile disputed the results.

In another National Cancer Institute research program letters were sent out to 835,000 doctors and 70,000 other health professionals. From this request there were found 67 patients whose results after taking Laetrile could be evaluated. The results were inconclusive, but because of the intense public interest in Laetrile, the National Cancer Institute is continuing the test. Supporters of Laetrile claim that these tests are biased and simply manifest the desire of the medical establishment to bury Laetrile. Medical critics of Laetrile claim that the cyanide contained in Laetrile is harmful to healthy cells. Supporters of Laetrile claim that the healthy cells are protected by another enzyme, rhodanase. Medical critics refute this claim.

What is the lay person to make of all this?

On the one hand, the medical establishment itself has been partly responsible for this conflict. It tends to reject possible therapies without a fair hearing simply because they have not come to its attention by the approved routing. A French Jesuit, Father Louis Beirnaent, has said, "We have spent too much time criticizing healers because they are not doctors and not enough time criticizing doctors who are not healers." The medical profession has at times, it seems, been rather paranoid in rejecting any kind of healing with which it was unfamiliar.

And although the stance of medical science today is

rigidly "scientific," as Dr. Herbert Benson of the Harvard Medical School has pointed out, until the latter part of the nineteenth century it was this same profession that subjected its patients to "purging, puking, poisoning, puncturing, cutting, cupping, blistering, bleeding, leeching, heating, freezing, sweating, and shocking." In the name of medical science, says Benson, "physicians have treated our battle wounds with boiling oil and red-hot pokers, have fed us lizard's blood, crushed spiders, crocodile dung, putrid meat, bear fat, fox lungs, eunuch fat, and moss scraped from the skull of a hanged criminal. Until recently, he concludes, "the physician's most potent tool in restoring his patient to good health" was the physician himself and his profound psychological effect upon the patient. Benson goes on to say that "it appears that medicine in the Western world, which was once an integration of both science and art, has shifted to an emphasis on science at the expense of art."

Perhaps the public response to the outlaw therapies for cancer, as well as other diseases, is partly a protest, both conscious and unconscious, against the dehumanization of the practice of medicine, a development against which many physicians themselves are striving. The wholistic health movement is directed toward restoring human values to health care, as well as toward the recognition that we are more than merely physical beings.

At the same time, the paranoia of some people in the medical profession is matched by a massive paranoia on the part of the lay public; the suspicion—in some cases, the obsession—that the medical establishment is trying to keep unorthodox cures from a fair trial. The result is that many people latch on to the outlaw therapies with a kind of religious commitment that refuses to be objective even in the face of evidence.

One of the objections of medical professionals to the outlaw therapies is that they deflect people from getting proper medical treatment. Often that is true and tragic. At the same time, however, there is a hollow ring to the charge that these are all fraudulent and criminal schemes to milk people of their money—particularly as some of the orthodox medical therapies have been largely unsuccessful and left their patients mutilated, bankrupt, and moribund. Vigilance against fraud is vital. But let us not brand all extramedical attempts at healing as fraudulent, especially for those who have been written off as medically hopeless.

In our own case, Valere and I were aware of many proclaimed cancer therapies. We did not find sufficient proof for any of them to be chosen as alternatives to orthodox medical procedures. At the same time, where we found no evidence of probable harm, we were willing to utilize any number of these so long as they did not seem to detract from the medical therapies we had selected.

We chose not to use the Hoxsey, Krebiozen, Kelley, or Laetrile* therapies. Some of the supplemental therapies we did utilize will be described in chapters nine and ten. None of these, we believe, detracted in any way from the best medical therapy we could find.

We believe that just as disease is the result of a complex of causes, so is healing multifaceted. As Christians, we believe that God is the source of all healing and uses many different means to accomplish that purpose—orthodox and unorthodox. Each person must make these choices for him or herself on the basis of the best information available. We believe in getting the best possible medical care, as well as utilizing anything else that seems likely to help rather than hurt.

One of these "anything else's" for us involved the possible healing power of the mind and spirit.

---

*For a discussion of Laetrile, see "In Defense of Laetrile," by Richard A. Passwater, *Let's Live Magazine,* June, 1977 *(pro);* and *The Breast,* by Oliver Cope, *(con),* pp. 122–26. Also chapter ten, "Experimental and Unproven Treatments," from *Choices,* by Morra and Potts *(pro* and *con).*

9. It's All in Your Mind

Mr. Wright was a patient with cancer of the lymph nodes.* His disease was so advanced that he did not even qualify for the test program of Krebiozen** at his hospital. The program stipulated that all participants have a life expectancy of from three to six months. Mr. Wright's physicians did not believe he was likely to live for another two weeks.

Mr. Wright was so excited about the Krebiozen research, however, that his physician, Dr. Philip West, reluctantly agreed to let him participate. Dr. West did not believe his patient would live long enough to receive his second dosage of Krebiozen in three days' time. "What a surprise was in store for me," relates Dr. West. "I had left him febrile, gasping for air, completely bedridden. Now,

*Mr. Wright's case reported by Bruno Klopfer in "Psychological Variables in Human Cancer," *Journal of Projective Techniques* (1957) pp. 337–39.

**Krebiozen was a substance developed in the early 1950s by two Yugoslavian brothers and advocated by Dr. Andrew Ivy, a professor of medical science who believed it to be effective in the treatment of cancer. Research to this date has not sustained his expectations.

here he was, walking around the ward, chatting happily with the nurses, and spreading his message of good cheer to any who would listen."

On the basis of Mr. Wright's reaction, Dr. West expected that other participants in the program would show similar improvement, but Mr. Wright proved to be the only patient with a positive response. Actually, Mr. Wright's progress was absolutely brilliant. "The tumor masses had melted like snowballs on a hot stove, and in only these few days they were half their original size!" Within ten days he was well enough to be discharged from his "deathbed, practically all signs of his disease having vanished in this short time." The "terminal" patient who had gasped for breath through an oxygen mask just a few days ago, now flew his own plane home at 12,000 feet with no discomfort!

Some time later, reports began to appear in the media indicating that the experiments with Krebiozen were meeting with disappointing results. When Mr Wright read these newspaper reports he began, after two months of practically perfect health, to experience a relapse. Soon he was back in the hospital, full of despair and cancer.

Dr. West was puzzled by Mr. Wright's response, both to the drug and to the reports in the media. Believing Mr. Wright had nothing to lose, he decided, as he puts it, to "play the quack." He told his patient that the newspapers had been in error and that the poor results they described had been the result of an inadequate dosage of the drug. He encouraged Mr. Wright to expect even better results from a dosage that would be twice as strong as before. "When I announced that the new series of injections was about to begin," reports Dr. West, "he was almost ecstatic and his faith was very strong."

With a deception that he thought was permissable under the circumstances, the physician began a second round of injections which were in reality nothing more than fresh water. Believing the injections to be an increased dosage of Krebiozen, Mr. Wright's recovery "was even more dramatic than the first. Tumor masses melted, chest fluid vanished, he became ambulatory, and even went back to flying again."

Once again Wright remained symptom-free for more than two months, until the final Americal Medical Association announcement appeared in the press—tests showed that Krebiozen was useless in the treatment of cancer. Within a few days of this report, Mr. Wright returned to the hospital. "His faith was now gone, his last hope vanished, and he succumbed in less than two days.

The phenomenon in Mr. Wright's case is hardly a common one in the annals of medicine. At the same time, it does happen. There is hardly a physician who has not experienced something similar at least once in his or her professional life. The medical profession calls these experiences *spontaneous remissions,* which is simply the profession's way of acknowledging that a patient has gotten well or significantly better for no known medical reason, often in defiance of existing medical science. Remissions may last a short time—as in Mr. Wright's case—or the patient may continue to defy medical odds and remain in a state of health.

Although these dramatic changes are called spontaneous, none of them really are. As Dr. Kenneth S. Pelletier has commented, "In each case there is some kind of cause-and-effect process." While a spontaneous remission may appear to be magical or miraculous (supernatural), it only appears to be so because we don't understand what forces are at work. Something is causing the dramatic change. If it defies normal medical science, it is only because "normal" experience is usually only a statistical average and there are a lot of possibilities that lie beyond the norm.

We might ascribe Mr. Wright's sudden recoveries—with tumors actually shrinking and melting away—to a sudden spurt of activity of his immune system. But obviously there was something else at work. It appears likely that this "something else" triggered powers of healing in Mr. Wright's own body that neither he nor his physician could have anticipated. It appears that that "something else" was his apparently mistaken faith in the healing power of Krebiozen. It is hard to escape the conclusion that Mr. Wright's own mind and spirit were able to call forth some physiological responses powerful enough to shrink and obliterate his cancerous tumor.

When Valere was diagnosed with breast cancer we both knew of Mr. Wright's case and of the healing power of the human mind/spirit in general. We knew and had been associated with Dr. O. Carl Simonton and his controversial use of mind power in the treatment of cancer. We had advocated and taught some of the same principles in our counselling and lectures.

Some of our friends thus wondered aloud why we were choosing any kind of medical therapy. "Why don't you go to Dr. Simonton?" they asked. It was a reasonable question, for Dr. Simonton's practice at that time was in Fort Worth, not far from Dallas. We did try to contact Dr. Simonton a number of times, but our attempts were unsuccessful, as he must have been out of town at the time and our messages apparently failed to reach him.

However, even if Valere had become Simonton's patient, it is doubtful that her therapy would have excluded orthodox medical treatment. Dr. Simonton himself would quite likely have prescribed radiation therapy. The use of the extramedical mind technique is not an alternative to orthodox medicine.

Because we were familiar with the extra medical techniques we felt quite confident about using them along with the program of radiation. And in fact, that's what we did. Today we are confident that these techniques, along with our religious faith, were supplementary and complementary to the radiation program. But that is a matter of belief, not fact.

Although we cannot prove that the powers of the mind and spirit were instrumental in Valere's healing, we know that there is substantial evidence that belief and faith are powerful factors in healing illness. Nor is this a phenomenon unknown in medical literature and clinical experience. Within the healing professions today day there is a dynamic movement known as the "wholistic" or "holistic" health approach. Kenneth Pelletier in his book *Mind as Healer, Mind as Slayer,* writes: "Holistic medicine recognizes the inextricable interaction between the person and his psychosocial environment. Mind and body function as an integrated unit, and health exists when they are in harmony, while illness results when stress and conflict disrupt this process."

Related to this approach is the concept of psychosomatic medicine, and attempt to understand both disease and health as the result of the interdependency and interplay of mind, body, and spirit. This means that the patient is not just a sick physical body—even less a single sick organ—but a dis-eased mind and spirit as well. The *psyche* is the mind/spirit dimension of the person and the *soma* is the body. Thus, *psychosomatic* means that both health and disease are affected by physical and psychic (mind/-spirit) factors.

Unfortunately, some people assume that psychosomatic means that a disease is imaginary. There were a few well-meaning friends who implied that Valere's breast cancer was "all in your mind." We knew, of course, that there was nothing imaginary about Valere's tumor. At the same time, we were not unaware that the physical disease had some mind/spirit perspectives.

We were already familiar with the books of Dr. Arnold Hutschnecker and his concepts linking physical disease with emotional states. "Illness," says Hutschnecker, "is the outer expression of a deep and possibly dangerous struggle going on within." Hutschnecker and others believe that an illness may be an unsconscious attempt to work out a conflict of some kind. Illness, therefore, may sometimes represent an unconscious desire to escape from a situation one does not want to cope with or is afraid he or she cannot handle. For example, it is not socially acceptable in our society for a person promoted to a higher position to acknowledge that he or she is inadequate to perform in that job. A heart attack, however, is perfectly acceptable and it achieves the same purpose.

Similarly, an illness may represent an unconscious strategy to control other people (and who can control a household more effectively than a demanding sick person?), to compensate for inadequate interpersonal relationships (the ulcer that can act as a substitute for love and affection is a good example), to work out feelings of anger, hostility, and bitterness, to inflict punishment upon one's self (and others), to list just a few.*

Several decades ago the German psychologist Dr. K. Marbe observed that for many people having accidents is no accident. These accident-prone people, he said, are motivated by an unconscious desire for punishment for a guilt they have not dealt successfully with on the conscious level. Dr. Karl Menninger of Kansas also believes that many people undergo surgery for the same reason: unconsciously to seek expiation from guilt by sacrificing a portion of their body.

So both accidents and illness may represent unconscious strategies for meeting frightening conflicts. In *Anatomy of an Illness,* Norman Cousins quotes Dr. Robert R. Rynearson: "As long as humans feel threatened and helpless, they will seek the sanctuary that illness provides."

Although the psychosomatic medicine and wholistic

*For further development of these ideas, see the author's book, *Rediscovering the Gift of Healing,* chapters 8, 9, 12. Nashville: Abingdon Press, 1977.

health movements are relatively new on the American medical scene, the concepts behind them are not. The healing shrines of Aescalapius, which eventually gave birth to the science of medicine, relied heavily upon the healing power of the mind/spirit. Hippocrates, the father of medicine, was very wholistic in his approach to disease and healing. Paracelsus understood, and his practice often reflected, psychosomatic principles, though the term itself was unknown at that time.

Dr. William Osler, considered the greatest clinician at the turn of the century, well understood and utilized what has come to be known as "the placebo effect." He believed that the cures of organic diseases under his care were due essentially not to the treatment he used, but to the patient's faith in the effectiveness of the treatment and to the comfort provided by good nursing care.

Nor is there anything new about the medical profession's use of the placebo. The placebo is a medication—usually a pill—which has no apparent medical value other than the patient's assumption that it will heal his disease or at least alleviate his symtoms. In the case of Mr. Wright the initial dosages of Krebiozen and later injections of water were placebos. That Mr. Wright nevertheless improved dramatically indicates that the healing power he attributed to the placebo was in his own mind. The placebo—inherently worthless—was effective because Mr. Wright had faith in it.

The medical profession often uses placebos in experimenting with drugs. Those participating are divided into three sub-groups: one that will not receive any medication, another that will receive a placebo, and a third that will be given the drug to be tested. By using this "double blind" method, the experimenters are assured that the result from the actual drug will be distinguishable from a placebo effect. When only two groups are used—one with the drug and one without—the experimenters can never be sure if positive effects are from the drug's healing qualities or a placebo effect, with the patient showing positive effects on the basis of his belief in the placebo. The placebo effect has been demonstrated again and again, proving the power of belief to effect cures or at least assist in the healing process. Dr. Herbert Benson, quotes New Zealand physician Dr. J.N.G. Davidson: "Let us remember, then, the power for good or for harm, not only of the drugs we put in our patients' bodies, but also—and of far greater importance—of the power for good, or harm, of the ideas and emotions we induce, wittingly or unwittingly, in our patients' minds."

Many physicians also attest to the power of a person's will to live. From a negative standpoint, Arnold Hutschnecker says, a patient who has a promising prognosis may die, not because he or she has consciously chosen to die, but because unconsciously the patient has not chosen to live. The will to live is a force that mobilizes the body's natural mechanisms of resistance to disease. Norman Cousins in his powerful testimony to the healing power of the mind/spirit, *Anatomy of an Illness,* tells us that one of the things he learned from his illness is that "the will to live is not a theoretical abstraction, but a physiologic reality with therapeutic characteristics. . . . I was incredibly fortunate to have as my doctor a man who knew that his biggest job was to encourage to the fullest the patient's will to live and to mobilize all the natural resources of body and mind to combat disease." Told by a specialist that his chances were one in five hundred and that he had not personally witnessed a patient recovering from the disease afflicting him, Cousins refused to accept this verdict and with his personal physician began a program that called for "the full exercise of the affirmative emotions as a factor in enhancing body chemistry." Among the features of that program was the "joyous discovery that ten minutes of genuine belly laughter had an anesthetic effect and would give me at least two hours of pain-free sleep."

Perhaps the best known—as well as the most controversial—program utilizing the healing powers of the mind/spirit has been developed by Dr. O. Carl Simonton and Stephanie Matthew-Simonton of Dallas, Texas. Simonton, an M.D., first developed some of his techniques while he was a naval physician in California. After his separation from the navy he moved to Fort Worth to practice oncology (the treatment of cancer) and test his ideas in earnest.

As a radiation oncologist, Dr. Simonton uses standard medical therapies—surgery, radiation, and chemotherapy—with techniques that have generally not been identified with cancer treatment. One facet of his program involves intensive counseling to help the patient gain awareness of his unconscious "insides" and to assist the patient in determining what role he or she has played in contracting the disease. Like Dr. Arnold Hutschnecker, whose works greatly influenced him, Dr. Simonton believes that the patient often unconsciously selects his or her disease, usually as a biological means to a psychological end: withdrawal, punishment, surrender to death, and so forth. Several years ago, at our house, Simonton was asked to speak to another dinner guest about the meaning of that guest's malignant brain tumor. He began with a shattering question: "What purpose do you think your brain tumor is serving?" Simonton believes that when the patient can acknowledge feelings and motivations, he or she is better able to fight the disease.

Another important feature of Simonton's extramedical program with the cancer patient involves the daily practice of relaxation-meditation. This technique is basically the progressive relaxation procedure pioneered by psychologist Edmund Jacobson. The purpose is both to physically relax the subject and to place him or her in a passive-receptive state of mind, similar to what is achieved with both bio-feedback and autogenic training.*

Relaxation and meditation techniques are being used by an increasing number of physicians and others to assist in treating various medical problems. In his book *The Relaxation Response* Dr. Herbert Benson has outlined the effectiveness of simple meditation in controling hypertension (high blood pressure) in his patients who were willing to learn the technique. Many of these were able to dispense with their hypertension medication.

Recently we encountered two medical doctors in the Dallas area—one a cardiologist, the other a general practitioner—who utilize meditation with some of their patients. According to Benson and these physicians, the physiological benefits of relaxation-meditation include a decrease in the pulse rate, blood pressure, and lactate concentration in the blood (both the galvanic skin response and high lactate concentrations are associated with states of anger and anxiety—what stress specialist Dr. Hans Selye calls "states of distress" the destructive rate of wear-and-tear on the body by excessive stress). Thus, any disease or physical condition that is stress-related may be treated at least in part by techniques of stress reduction, of which relaxation-meditation is one of the most effective.

In addition to intensive counseling and relaxation-meditation technique Simonton uses visualization or imagery to gain control over certain autonomic (unconsciously directed) functions of the body. Bio-feedback has repeatedly demonstrated that people may learn to avoid

*Bio-feedback is the use of monitoring equipment to help the subject learn to gain conscious control over normally unconscious bodily functions: respiration rate, heartbeat, brain-wave patterns, and so forth. Autogenic training is a technique developed by German psychiatrist Johannes H. Schultz in the 1930s to accomplish much the same thing without machine feedback.

or cancel migraine headaches, reduce stomach acidity, and ward off attacks of epilepsy—to name just a few conditions—utilizing the usually undeveloped powers of the mind over the body. Similar results have been achieved with meditation and autogenic training, which also employ visualization techniques.

Dr. Simonton believes that we can also learn to control or influence the body's immune system, which is an autonomous system in the human organism. For example, a patient with leukemia is encouraged to visualize this scenario: a large red army engages and overwhelms a white army—the red army symbolizing the blood's red cells which need to overcome the cancerous white cells. Practicing this visualization several times daily, Simonton believes, is a valuable therapy in fighting leukemia. It is based upon the body's inherent capacities for overcoming disease; visualization is simply a technique to mobilize those capacities. (In a sense it may not be extramedical at all when we contemplate that much of medical science today is based upon the mobilization of those same capacities through the use of chemicals and other means.)

In 1974 I invited Dr. Simonton to Calvary United Methodist Church in Mohnton, Pennsylvania, to speak about his work and show slides illustrating some of the dramatic results he was experiencing in his work. Among those which he shared with us were these:

—A thirty-eight-year-old man with a cancer growth the size of a walnut lodged in his throat enthusiastically followed the Simonton program (orthodox medical treatment plus the three-fold extramedical techniques). Ten weeks later he saw X-ray evidence that the cancerous tissue has been replaced by normal tissue.

—A fifty-five-year-old woman with a large, advanced anal cancer was completely well in six weeks. X rays three years later show only a slight loss of pigment in the skin.

—A twelve-year-old boy with a very large scrotal cancer experienced a dramatic shrinkage of the cancer in two weeks.

While some physicians and psychologists have criticized Simonton's published data and are skeptical of his claims, similar results have been reported by others.* Dr. Jeanne Achterberg and G. Frank Lawlis, a husband and wife psychology team in Dallas, Texas, have published their findings in two books, *Imagery of Cancer* and *Bridges of the Bodymind.*** Many of their studies have focused on the technique of imagery. One of their findings: there is

---

*A Circular Letter dated August 28, 1981, from the American Cancer Society (specifically from the Vice President for Professional Education), titled "Unproven Methods of Cancer Management—'O. Carl Simonton, M.D.,'" states that the consensus of two independently conducted studies by Departments of Psychiatry at Memorial–Sloan Kettering Cancer Center and Mt. Sinai Hospital in New York City is that "Dr. Simonton's position is believed to be untenable in treatment of cancer patients from a psychological and psychosomatic point of view and scientific data does not support his arguments. In addition, real potential hazards for patients are associated with induction of guilt feelings, overreliance on the Simonton technique, and with abandonment of generally accepted treatments, in spite of Dr. Simonton's advice to continue them."

It is regrettable that this ACS paper seems primarily directed at "shooting down" Simonton, instead of dealing with other studies which, although not *proof* of the mind-body cancer link, are at least *evidence* that must be dealt with before a final verdict can be pronounced. Some medical doctors, psychiatrists, and psychologists believe that that evidence is most persuasive. The mindbody link has been successfully demonstrated in numerous other diseases. Why should it be so unthinkable with cancer? The American Cancer Society Circular Letter on this subject is probably as "scientific," "fair" and "final" as its similar pronouncement on the use of irradiation in the treatment of breast cancer given to us by Dr. Jowl.

**Dr. Lawlis is Associate Professor of Psychology at North Texas State University and Associate Professor of Physical Medicine at the University of Texas Health Science Center in Dallas. Dr. Achterberg is Assistant Professor of Physical Medicine at the Center in Dallas.

a statistical relationship between the types of images patients use and the outcome of their disease or rehabilitation. Inasmuch as imagery is reflective of the unconscious mind, this would seem to be another link between the unconscious and physical disease and recuperation.

Other researchers who have responded favorably to the extramedical approach include Dr. Bernard Siegel, a New Haven, Connecticut, surgeon, Dr. Ronald Waggener at Methodist Hospital in Omaha, Nebraska, and Dr. Rick Ingrasci in Newton, Massachusetts.

"We've been doing the same thing for years," Dr. Elmer Green of the Menninger Foundation in Topeka, Kansas, told us recently (August, 1981). Actually, said Dr. Green, the techniques are not all that mysterious, for visualization simply invokes the body's own self-regulation effect, of which the placebo effect—a phenomenon known to every medical doctor—is merely a subdivision. When a general practitioner gives a patient a chemically worthless sugar pill for some real or imagined condition, he is inducing the patient to visualize a cure or relief. The placebo effect, Dr. Green says in *Beyond Bio-Feedback* (written with Alyce Green), works only with organisms that can be induced to visualize. "That's why you don't have a placebo effect with babies and dogs." Visualization, therefore, is a means of gaining conscious control over the body's own self-regulation systems.

If, as many researchers have demonstrated, the mind triggers various neurological and chemical responses in the body, ultimately impinging on a person's health, it seems no less reasonable to believe that the mind may be similarly used to trigger neurological and endocrinological reactions that affect the body's own natural resource system capacity to heal itself or maintain health.

Valere devised a number of visualization meditations for the period of her irradiation therapy and in the recuperation period afterward. Here are some of the visualization scenarios she used:

• While she was waiting her turn for radiation therapy, Valere visualized a "healing light" which pervaded her whole being and everyone in the waiting room. She devised this particular visualization because she was afraid she would become depressed as she sat among many patients with advanced cancer. This technique enabled her to remain positive and hopeful in what otherwise would have been a very draining atmosphere.

• When she entered the room to receive her daily radiation treatment she used both an affirmation and a visualization. The affirmation was: "I am receiving the correct amount of radiation and it is being focused upon the precise place where it is needed." She visualized her cancer cells being bombarded with pellets of light that completely obliterated the cancerous growth. The room to which she was taken each day for radiation was "scary," because of the size of the radiation machine and because the technicians were so careful to avoid exposure themselves to the radiation. She felt the technique made her more receptive to the radiation treatment and helped eliminate some of the emotional barriers that might have been a negative factor.

• Whenever Valere ate a meal during the period of radiation therapy, she both affirmed and visualized that the food she was eating provided the necessary nutrition for her recovery. This may be one reason why, despite warnings that radiation therapy might suppress her appetite, she maintained a healthy appetite throughout the entire five-week procedure.

• Whenever she urinated, she visualized the dead cancer cells being expelled from her body. This was one of the easiest visualizations because it was used simultaneously with a physiological function.

• At random times during the day, she visualized herself

at the very peak of her health and vitality. This involved mind pictures of considerable physical activity and a pervasive feeling of great well-being.

· At least three times per day she went through a complete relaxation-meditation and visualized a scenario in which, at a considerably advanced age (eighties), she saw herself standing before a large audience telling of her successful treatment for cancer of the breast many years previous.

· An affirmation which she randomly repeated at various times during the day was: "All things are possible with God."

She recorded some of these affirmations and visualization scenarios on cassette tapes before she went to the hospital for her implants. When she was in isolation for the implants, she played these tapes over and over and although she sometimes felt lonely, she never experienced any despair or worry.*

These are merely some of the means Valere employed to keep herself in a positive, receptive state of mind during the radiation therapy and the weeks that followed. How can we measure the effectiveness of these techniques as they relate to her process of healing? We cannot, and our conviction of their positive contribution is a subjective response. That does not mean that we are any less convinced of their efficacy.

What possible positive effects can these techniques have? We know that certain negative emotions call forth certain specific physiological responses. For example, fear releases adrenalin into the bloodstream. Anger releases noradrenalin. We do not know why one emotion provokes one neurochemical response, while a different emotion

---

*Copies of these tapes are available from the New Dimensions Center, First United Methodist Church, Ross & Harwood Sts., Dallas, Texas 75201.

provokes another. But we do know that there is a direct link between certain emotional states and specific neurochemical reactions in the body. We think it entirely likely that, in the same manner, certain positive emotional states provoke the release of other neurochemical reactions which are beneficial to restoring or maintaining health.

We also believe that Valere's positive, hopeful state of mind contributed in some degree to her receptivity to the radiation therapy. It may well be that such an emotional climate provokes in some patients a positive response to a therapy, while in others there is a distinct negative result.

No one quite understands how this may operate, but one possible clue is in the working of the unconscious mind. The affirmations and the imagery do have an effect upon the unconscious mind which is control of the various autonomic operations of the body systems. Some of the techniques are nothing less than an attempt to impress the unconscious with a concept that the conscious mind is not capable of making operative in the life of the individual. For example, Dr. Achterberg and G. Frank Lawlis found that "what the patient may say [and intellectually believe] outwardly about an illness and its treatment may not reflect unconscious or innermost feelings. . . . You can ask a patient if he thinks he will get well," says Dr. Achterberg. "He may say yes, but his imagination [as evidenced in his iamgery] may not reflect unconscious or innermost feelings."

This does not mean that the development of cancer is either imaginary or automatic. Certain emotional states trigger various chemical reactions in the body. It has been proven that prolonged states of depression or despair often affect the body's hypothalamic and pituitary activity. The result may be a suppression of the immune system and an imbalance in the endocrine system that can contribute to the increase of abnormal cells. Emotional stress inadequately handled does not automatically cause cancer, but it may very well contribute to the causes.

In a similar manner, the use of psychological or spiritual intervention does not automatically cure cancer. However, by changing both our perceptions of ourselves and our problems (often through creative imagination, belief, faith, and so forth), we may also positively affect hypothalamic and pituitary activity, increasing immune system functioning and restoring hormonal balance—thus contributing to the regression and even cure of cancer. In short, these methods may contribute to the conditions that *allow* recovery to take place.

As mentioned earlier, the extramedical techniques have drawn skepticism and severe criticism. One aspect of that criticism will be dealt with in the next chapter. As Constance Holden has observed in *Science Magazine*, "Clearly it's going to be a while before biochemical research establishes the role of the mind in precipitating cancer, or of that ill-defined but potent factor—the will to live—in mobilizing physical defenses once the disease has set in. Nonetheless, for a growing cadre of people involved in the psychological treatment of cancer victims, the evidence, while not definitive, is enough."

We thought so then and we are even more certain now—so long as these techniques are regarded as a supplemental therapy and not an alternative to orthodox medical treatment, so long as disciples of the technique do not make a cult of the technique and surround it with dogmatic demands for a religious type of commitment.

Dr. Bernard Siegel, a general surgeon affiliated with the Yale New Haven Hospital and Hospital St. Raphael's, New Haven, Connecticut, has been using some of these extramedical techniques since 1978, including guided imagery (visualization), relaxation-meditation, and counseling that attempts to enable the patient to participate in his/her treatment. Dr. Siegel told us (October, 1980) that when he began his extra medical program, local physicians were hostile, indifferent, or curious. Now, however, he says an increasing number of physicians are referring patients to him. Siegel and his associates believe there has been a measurable positive difference in the medical progress of a majority of the more than 150 people who have passed through his program. Some physicians have changed their attitudes about Siegel's program, he says, because they have witnessed that participants appear to respond more favorably to chemotherapy, radiation, and other medical therapies.

There is another aspect of the mind/spirit perspective on cancer that we utilized during Valere's period of treatment and recovery: the healing power of a strong support system. Our particular support strategy included making the most of our spiritual and religious resources. Without asking, we were assured by scores of friends across the country that they were holding Valere in prayer, which was for us a very meaningful assurance. I did my best to surround her with a positive, constructive healing environment. In some cases, we simply avoided people whose reaction to her cancer was negative and depressive. I had long ago discovered that some people, when they learn that a friend or associate has contracted cancer, will unconsciously begin to speak of the patient in the past tense: "Poor John, he was such a great guy!" I was determined to keep Valere from that kind of influence, no matter how well intentioned. Furthermore, we programmed our lives during the period of radiation treatment to be in contact with as many stimulating and positive people as we knew. Our sightseeing and visiting during this period was consciously designed to be as upbeat as possible.

Secondly, I encouraged Valere to the degree that she felt able to continue working. Since she was self-employed, this was no great problem. I felt she should not sit around and worry or feel sorry for herself. Perhaps I was not always so wise in not restraining her work when she was at a low physical ebb, but if we had to err on one side or another, I preferred that it be on the side of doing too much.

Since Valere's treatment and recovery, we have since learned of a number of organized support groups in throughout the United States. I've already mentioned the two programs for mastectomy patients, the American Cancer Society's Reach to Recovery and the YWCA's Encore. There are other programs: one started by Don Gilley (himself the recipient of a remarkable cure following the Simonton program) in Charlotte, North Carolina, called Dayspring; Orville Kelley's Make Today Count with headquarters in Burlington, Iowa (Kelley was also a cancer patient); the American Cancer Society's Cansurmount and I Can Cope; the Rev. Thomas A. Welch's Focus in Cambridge, Massachusetts; and New York's Living With Cancer. Our own New Dimensions Center affiliated with First United Methodist Church in Dallas, Texas, also attempts to provide assistance to cancer patients.

The National Cancer Institute has been so impressed with the importance of support groups that it funded a study of 800 patients who had mastectomies, colostomies, or laryngectomies. Theresa Rogers, a sociologist at Columbia University, has been their principal investigator. Another study is being conducted at UCLA to determine the effect of self-help groups on the outcome of treatment in patients with life-threatening diseases. Iris Pearce is conducting two of the UCLA projects, including a group of thirty patients, twenty-two of whom are still alive after being informed that they had but one year to live. Another organization that has been active in assisting cancer patients in mobilizing their full resources is the New Wineskins Center connected with the First Community Church in Columbus, Ohio.

We believe that any methods or programs that can mobilize our human resources to co-operate in the treatment of cancer and which do not conflict with proven orthodox cancer therapies are worth the time and effort we may invest in them.

That, at least, was our experience.

Valere's cancer was certainly not all in her mind. Neither was her healing all in her body.

10. An Ounce of Prevention

This chapter is written for

—those who have *not* had breast cancer, and . . .

—those who *have* had breast cancer.

In short, the prevention of breast cancer is a vital subject for all women. *Prevention,* as we're using it here, means what you can do to reduce your risk of ever having breast cancer and the steps you can take to minimize serious illness if you do have a malignancy in the breast. Breast cancer, when diagnosed early, is least difficult to treat successfully.

If we are going to work at preventing breast cancer, it is important that we take a look at some of the factors which may be responsible for this disease.

What Is the Cause of Breast Cancer?

As already described, breast cancer cells are normal cells that go haywire and begin to behave in a manner quite at odds with the way they were designed to function. The cancer cell becomes locked into a cycle of almost constant growth and division and will likely invade cells and tissues adjacent to it, scavenging off their nutrients and resources. But what causes the cancer cell to do these things? A partial answer seems to be that there has been some malfunction in its genetic information. It is an imperfect cell. But that still leaves us with the questions as to why it is imperfect; what has caused it to malfunction?

This time the answer is a simple one: no one really knows. You may be sure that if we knew the precise cause of breast cancer we would be a lot closer to an effective cure. However, although no one has scientifically proven what causes breast cancer, there is a lot of evidence that suggests several different answers, none of which need exclude the others.

Among those most likely are the following:

Carcinogenics

A carcinogenic is any substance—usually chemical—which is likely to cause cancer. Our knowledge of likelihood that a substance is carcinogenic is determined pretty much through the testing of animals. When these animals have been exposed to large dosages of a suspected carcinogenic agent over a period of time and the incidence of cancer rises significantly, the agent is tabbed as carcinogenic or cancer-producing. Among these substances most commonly identified as carcinogenics are asbestos, aniline dyes, coal tars, food colors and preservatives, artificial sweeteners, and other chemicals. Almost every week there is a report about some newly discovered carcinogenic agent—usually something that you and I have been using with some frequency. Sometimes these reports are challenged by other researchers who claim that exposing laboratory mice to large amounts of certain substances doesn't prove that these items in moderate amounts are carcinogenic to human beings.

In December, 1978, we read a newspaper story with the headline, "Cancer Chief Wary of Some Hair Dyes." Dr. Arthur Upton was quoted as advising consumers to stop using hair dyes containing a chemical known as 4-methoxy-m-phenylenediamine or 2-4 diaminoanisole. We wrote the Clairol Corporation, manufacturers of about half the hair dyes in the United States, to inquire if this chemical was contained in their products. Back came a two-page letter from Arnetha Matthews, "Consultant," who informed me that it was not being used by Clairol, citing a string of research projects by various reputable groups that proved Clairol's products to be safe. There was also included a printed statement from the Cosmetic, Toiletry, and Fragrance Association along the same lines.

One year later, February, 1979, another story appeared in the paper indicating that researchers at the New York University's Institute of Environmental Medicine in a study published in the *Journal of the National Cancer Institute* had found that "breast cancer in women older than fifty may be linked to prolonged use of hair dyes." The article also noted that the Cosmetic, Toiletry, and Fragrance Association had attacked the new study and that Clairol had "dropped three suspected cancer-causing chemicals from its hair dyes last year after the U.S. Food & Drug Administration proposed a warning label for one of them."

To date so far as we have been able to determine, this dispute has not been resolved. Agencies such as the American Cancer Society and the National Cancer Institute have not issued policy statements on this subject.

So where does that leave us if we are concerned in preventing breast cancer? It leaves us with the possibility that some hair dye chemicals may be carcinogenic but there is no proof and evidence is conflicting at best.

One of the things we need to remember about these kinds of statistics is that they are not hard proof. On a broad statistical basis involving large numbers of people, it is evident that there is an increased incidence of cancer when people are exposed to certain substances. At the same time, there are great numbers of people who are exposed and still do not contract cancer. There are also people who are exposed to small amounts of carcinogens and do contract the disease. What this means is that exposure to carcinogens is not the sole answer.

Therefore, a carcinogen may be only one of a number of factors that may cause cancer. Since many are exposed and do not get cancer, we must decide on the basis of evidence available if we will cut down on our exposure to a particular substance or eliminate it entirely. If a person has already had one incidence of cancer, it would seem wise to reduce exposure to known carcinogens as much as possible.

Diet

There is even less certainty and proof when we examine the relationship of diet and breast cancer. In general, the medical profession holds that there is no proof of a causative relationship between diet and breast cancer. Some in the medical community believe, however, that there is some evidence for a link. Furthermore, a fair number of nutritionists believe that they have proven that nutrition and dietary management can both prevent and assist in curing cancer of the breast.

At a National Breast Cancer Teach-In sponsored by the American Cancer Society in September, 1979, Dr. Ernst Wynder, President of the American Health Foundation and the scientist who tied cigarette smoking to lung cancer, said that he believes there is considerable evidence, although not fully proven, to indicate that people with a high fat diet are more likely to develop cancer, including cancer of the breast. He based his conclusions on patterns of distribution of breast cancer throughout the world, which indicate a significantly higher incidence where the diet is high in fats; laboratory tests with rats which show that a high-fat diet produces increased levels of prolactin, a pituitary hormone linked to cancer; studies of women with a late first pregnancy (after age twenty-six) indicating high prolactin levels which can be reduced with low-fat diets. Wynder called for a diet low in all fats—animal, vegetable, polyunsaturated, and saturated.

Dr. Wynder and others believe that the low fat content in the diet may account for the significantly lower incidence of breast cancer among Japanese women than in American women. It has also been noticed that women of Japanese ancestry in the United States have a higher incidence of breast cancer than women in Japan, pointing perhaps to a dietary rather than a genetic factor. Although most cancer authorities have not hurried to endorse this view officially, a survey of a number of "leading cancer doctors" in the United States, as reported by Jean McCann in the *Medical Tribune*, revealed that many of them, when asked what they personally did to prevent cancer, listed a low-fat diet as part of their own regimen.

Other physicians believe that a high caloric intake may be linked to cancer on the basis of experiments with laboratory animals. Some believe that overweight may also be a factor and, in the McCann survey, Dr. Arthur Holleb, director of medical affairs of the American Cancer Society, said "there's a strong relationship between obesity and breast cancer."

A number of nutritionists—normally outside the medical establishment—believe that there is evidence for an even stronger link between breast cancer and nutrition. One of the leading spokesmen for this point of view is Carleton Fredericks, a nutritionist associated with the International Academy of Preventive Medicine. Noting that one-third of all breast cancers are estrogen-dependent (a term explained in chapter eight), Dr. Fredericks claims that certain dietary practices can prevent cancer and even help cure it. He also disputes high-fat diet as the nutritional culprit, noting that "the American black female consumes more fat than her white counterpart, but has less breast cancer," and that other ethnic groups such as the Eskimo, Mongolian, and Massai (Africa) women have diets very high in fat and at the same time very little, if any, cancer.

Dr. Fredericks's program is focused on the dietary control of the body's own production of estrogen through the use of inositol (a B-complex vitamin), the reduction of sugar intake, adequate amounts of protein, and vitamin B-complex. Fredericks also advocates high dosages of vitamin C—or at least dosages in excess of government-recommended minimum levels, which he believes are disastrously low.

Dr. Fredericks also makes the startling charge: "There is a .64 correlation between sugar consumption and breast cancer, meaning that 64 times in every 100, you will find a higher incidence of the disease associated with higher intake of sweets." Unfortunately, Fredericks does not cite a source for that statistic.*

Critics of the nutritionists' claims concerning diet and cancer have noted that one of the nation's most popular and well-read nutritionists, Adelle Davis, died of cancer in 1974 at the age of seventy. If nutrition is so effective in preventing cancer, they asked, why did one of the nation's top nutritionists die of the very disease she said could be prevented by good nutrition? In an article for *New Woman*, nutritionist George E. Berkley attempted to answer the critics by suggesting that Adelle Davis not only didn't follow some of her own nutrition principles, but was also wrong in some others—errors that made her susceptible to cancer. So, it seems, "you pays your money and you takes your choice." Unfortunately there is too little agreement among the experts. For the most part, the medical

---

*For a full explanation of Fredericks's views, see his book, *Winning the Fight Against Breast Cancer: The Nutritional Approach.* New York: Grosset & Dunlap, 1977.

establishment has paid little attention to diet and nutrition in the cure and prevention of breast cancer. There seems to be a move toward change in that regard, but much research is necessary before these questions can be settled.

There are also many dietary "cures" for breast cancer. Some people advocate an asparagus diet, while others recommend almonds. While Valere was undergoing radiation therapy, friends suggested that she take chaparral, a substance taken from a plant that grows in areas of the southwest, which is reputed to be the primary reason for the low incidence of of cancer in Indians living in these areas. Taken as a tea or tablet, chaparral is reputed to be effective in purging the body of poisons. While there were anecdotal testimonies concerning its effectiveness, we found no proof. But, since it is not expensive and there seemed to be no bad effects from taking it, we decided it couldn't hurt and it might help. We still don't know what, if any, benefit Chaparral may have had.

There is evidence that proper diet and nutrition may be helpful in the prevention and treatment of breast cancer. Since the reduction of fat in the diet is recommended as beneficial to health on a number of grounds and the reduction of sugar intake is similarly recommended across the board, these would be wise moves in any case. If a person has had at least one incident of cancer, it would seem foolish not to make some dietary changes that, although not necessarily proven to be effective, appear to be beneficial according to available evidence. Carleton Fredericks's program appears to be relatively inexpensive, easy, and safe.

The problem with any program of prevention, of course, is that you are only acutely aware of its failure. Good health is hard to measure and even harder to attribute to something specific.

As in the case of carcinogens, diet is probably one

factor, but not *the* factor or single cause in breast cancer.*

Genetic Factors

We are told that a woman has a greater chance for getting breast cancer if her mother or sister, or both, have had a breast malignancy. Thus it is believed that the predisposition to cancer is something that is passed along to some women in their genes. Although genetic factors are used in identifying women who are in a high-risk category for breast cancer, medical professionals believe that it is only one of several factors that may be operative in the incidence of breast cancer.

We need to remember, therefore, that a family history of breast cancer does not doom a woman to that disease. At the most, it increases her statistical risk. Obviously, many women—a majority actually—whose mother or sister had breast cancer do not contract breast cancer themselves.

Radiation

Another suspected cause of cancer is radiation. We know that radiation can cause mutations in cells and that mutations are related to cancerous growths. We know also that excessive exposure to the sun directly increases the incidence of skin cancers (which are really quite different from breast cancers). Some experts also believe that the release of flourocarbons (from aerosol spray cans) have been responsible for destroying a protective layer of ozone in the earth's atmosphere, thus leading to an increased exposure to ultraviolet radiation from the sun.

---

*For a recent source on nutritional aspects of cancer, see *Jane Brody's Nutrition Book* by Jane Brody, New York: W.W. Norton, 1981.

Physicians have also disputed the role of excessive exposure to X rays and other kinds of radiation (from TV sets, microwave ovens, and so forth). Some surgeons have expressed concern that radiation therapy may be responsible for increased rates of cancer. Radiologists have countered those claims with the argument that statistics from radiation therapy do not substantiate those fears.

Valere was invited to represent a patient's point of view on a panel of physicians in New York, on October 15, 1980, under the auspices of the American College of Radiology. One of the reporters present asked whether anyone had computed the long-term chances of a radiation-induced tumor as a result of breast irradiation. Dr. Luther Brady, one of the panel members, replied that this was not a concern with the dosage that is given in breast irradiation —5,000 rads delivered with high energy accelerators over a period of five weeks. He went on to say: "Long-term observation of thousands and thousands of patients indicates that the risk for radiation-induced cancer in that particular group is not increased over what it would have been had the breast never been irradiated. So, the potential is minimal at worst and probably none at best."

But the reporter wanted to take his question one step further: "All right, let me make sure I understand this. Now, if you take mammography, would you see a slightly increased risk of cancer just from that?"

This time the answer came from Dr. Samuel H. Madell, the moderator of the panel and a professor of radiology at Albert Einstein College of Medicine in New York: "No. That's not so. There is no known or observed increase in cancer incidence from any diagnostic radiologic procedure at all. . . . There is no known biologic effect on humans by radiation in the dose levels of diagnostic examinations. No known or or ever-observed effect. Nevertheless, there are effects at higher doses. Therefore it is said that it might be prudent to suppose that there might be similar effects over a long-range of time for smaller doses. It's all extrapolated. There is no scientific knowledge."

So, the mammogram does carry with it some risk, but it is a risk that has not been demonstrated except by mathematical projection. As a result, the National Cancer Institute, the American College of Radiology, and the American Cancer Society have developed guidelines for the use of mammograms for screening and diagnosis:

Women over 50: annual screening recommended (since benefits clearly outweigh minimal long-term risk)

Women 35–50: screening recommended for women in the following high-risk categories:
chronic cystic mastitis
lumps and thickening in the breast
nipple discharge or other nipple abnormalities
personal history of breast cancer
family history of breast cancer (maternal, paternal, or sisters)
early onset of menstruation
no previous pregnancy
first fulltime pregnancy at age thirty or older
breast surgery scheduled for diagnostic purposes
fear of breast cancer that requires reassurance by negative examination

(It is estimated that 80 percent of the women in the 35–50 group will fit into one of these ten categories.)

Women 35–50: self-examination for those who do not fit into the high-risk categories above

Women under 35: self-examination if without breast problems

Because mammography helps to identify breast cancers at a considerably earlier stage than self- or physician-examination, the benefits far outweigh the theoretical risks. As Dr. Luther Brady has said in his presidential address to the American Radium Society: "An unsuspected cancer, successfully treated, is a medical triumph." Dr. Brady reported that for cancers detected by mammography alone, five-year survival rates of up to 95 percent have been reported. So the benefit of early detection by the mammogram is a real one, while the risk is theoretical.

As in the case of radiation therapy, the technology of mammography has also greatly improved. Recent monitoring shows that a woman's breast will absorb less than one rad in the average mammogram performed at National Cancer Institute/American Cancer Society centers.

To this must be added the following factor: many people who have been exposed to high levels of radiation, X ray and otherwise, do not get cancer, while others whose exposure has been minimal do get it. Radiation may be a factor in cancer, but it is hardly *the* cause.

Estrogen/the Pill

As has already been discussed, approximately one-third of all malignant breast tumors are dependent upon or responsive to the estrogen hormone. It would be reasonable to conclude that at least some breast cancers may be caused by excessive hormone levels and therefore that the use of the contraceptive pill as well as estrogen supplements may be dangerous. Nevertheless, few physicians have taken this position. Dr. Marvin Kirschner of the New Jersey Medical School in Newark reported to the 1976 White House Conference on Breast Cancer that on the basis of hormone studies to date, "it is apparent that in spite of tantalizing bits of data linking breast cancer development with possible alteration of endocrine function, no clear-cut or comprehensible patterns are yet evident."

Dr. Phillip Strax, whose book, *Early Detection: Breast Cancer Is Curable,* is distributed in a condensed form by the American Cancer Society, says: "There is no definite evidence so far to incriminate 'the pill' in the development of breast cancer, although some experts have doubts about the pill. The truth is that it will take another ten years before we may know definitely whether or not such pills are harmful."

Still, Dr. Strax himself must have some doubts, for he added: "Women on 'the pill' definitely should have a complete breast examination at least once a year." Every doctor who examined Valere before her lumpectomy and irradiation routinely asked if she was on the pill or taking any estrogen supplements. Every doctor also instructed her—not advised—to cease all estrogen supplements immediately. And at least one of them could not hide his surprise—registered with arched eyebrows—when he learned she had been on premarin (estrogen) for more than fifteen years and exceptionally high dosages had been prescribed by her gynecologist since her hysterectomy a few years previous.

Although a major study in 1975 linked breast cancer and estrogen, three additional studies since then have both supported and attacked those findings. No wonder the lay public is confused and the medical profession can't agree! For the time being, perhaps the most we can conclude is this: Given the apparent risks in the use of estrogen supplements, those women who have had an incidence of cancer are wise to discontinue them completely; those who have not had cancer but are in higher-risk categories would do well to give discontinuance careful consideration.

Other Causes?

One thing about which the entire medical profession seems to be in complete agreement is that breast cancer is not caused by sexual activity, including excessive (whatever that is) handling or fondling of the breasts. Roughness in handling the breast may cause pain, and even bruises, but not cancer, say the doctors.

The medical people seem equally in agreement that other traumas or blows to the breast do not cause breast cancer. We had been somewhat concerned on this score, for just one year prior to the discovery of Valere's cancer, she had had a blow to the breast while we were in a Land Rover in Sri Lanka. Although all physicians assured us there was no connection with her malignancy, we have been intrigued by the number of other breast-cancer patients who report similar breast traumas prior to the discovery of their disease.

Geography and climate are not believed to affect the incidence of breast cancer, although the rate is certainly higher in some states than others, and the incidence among urban women is higher than among those in rural areas. We have already reported significant differences in the incidence among Japanese and other oriental women and American women. Similarly, women in highly industrialized nations run a substantially greater risk. One interesting finding is that there is significantly less breast cancer among Mormons and even less among Seventh Day Adventists. Although the reasons have not been identified, the leading interpretation seems to relate to dietary differences. Also Mormons and Seventh Day Adventists have a different lifestyle in which stress and emotions may be managed in a more successful manner.

We have already noted that some people in the medical field attribute the onset of cancer in general and breast cancer in particular to a malfunction or overpowering of the body's own immune system. Why is it that most people whose family has a history of cancer, or who are exposed to carcinogens, radiation, and high-fat diets remain healthy? In his book, Dr. Simonton answers that "the development of a cancer does not require just the presence of abnormal cells; it also requires *a suppression of the body's normal defenses.*"

Dr. Simonton and others believe that we are frequently subjected to cancerous cells, but when the immune system is working at its optimum, the cancers are eliminated without our awareness—just as many of us have had undiscovered bouts with the TB bacillus and, apart from scar tissue on our lungs, are unaware of it.

This is sometimes called the *surveillance theory*, which holds that the body's immune system normally keeps the body under surveillance for abnormal cells and destroys them. The cancerous growth occurs, according to this theory, when the immune system has in some way been inhibited. Once again, unfortunately, we are in an area of considerable disagreement. Some physicians discount this theory and one cancer specialist, Dr. Paul Calabresi, chairman of the Department of Medicine at Brown University and Roger Williams Hospital in Providence, Rhode Island, told us recently that a number of findings in the past five to ten years have contributed to the decline in popularity of the surveillance theory. These findings do not dispute the role of the body's own immune system, but indicate that the operation of that system is much more complex than was first believed. It is too simplistic, Dr. Calabresi said, to assume that cancer is the mere result of some failure in the immune system.

This dispute over the surveillance theory does not necessarily threaten to invalidate the mind-over-body or psychosomatic approaches, but it does mean that the operation of the immune system is likely to be only one factor in the incidence of disease. The system does not operate with the mechanical certainty and omnipotence that was once ascribed to it.

Nevertheless, there seems to be considerable evidence that links illness with the way we handle stress. This has been demonstrated not only in laboratory tests with animals, but also with human beings as well.

The pioneer in charting the causes and effects of excessive stress is Dr. Hans Selye, an Austrian physician who now resides and works in Canada. His work has persuaded members of the medical profession to believe that inappropriate handling of stress may open the body's physical defenses to invasion by disease-causing agents. Among these are cancer-producing antigens. If this is so, and the evidence is persuasive, then one preventive for cancer in general and breast cancer in particular would be to deal creatively with stress in our daily lives.

Convinced of the validity of this approach, Valere and I have worked constantly on the techniques of stress management in our own lives. These techniques include self-discovery and understanding, meditation, bio-feedback, and autogenic training. For the person who has already suffered one affliction with cancer or the person in a high-risk category, we believe stress management may be an effective means of prevention.

Beyond the destructive effects of stress and other mind/body factors, there are some who believe that a certain personality type is more likely to be susceptible to cancer. The keystone of this approach has been the work of Dr. Lawrence LeShan, a New York clinical psychologist. Dr. LeShan was asked to work with a group of terminal cancer patients. His object was to help them deal more effectively with their emotional reactions to their disease, and thus improve the quality of the time remaining to them. Dr. LeShan was successful in helping them to make a more positive adjustment to their disease and impending death. On this basis alone, the project would have been deemed most successful. But two other things occurred that LeShan had not anticipated: some of the patients, after having dealt with the serious emotional conflicts in their lives in their sessions with him, experienced remarkable remissions in their cancer—and some even failed to die. LeShan concluded that if emotional factors may cause or contribute to the contraction of cancer, resolving emotional conflicts may cure the disease or at least bring some remission. Dr. Simonton and others have structured their use of psychotherapy according to this premise.

As a result of this project, LeShan also noted the emergence of what he came to regard as a "cancer personality profile." He found that the majority of cases had personality factors and structures that were common, if not identical. On the basis of these findings and work with additional groups, LeShan developed a cancer personality profile that looks like this:

—a person who has lost his or her reason for being

—a person who is unable to express anger or resentment adequately

—a person who suffers from some degree of self-dislike or self-distrust

—a person who suffers a high degree of despair (a despair that exists in the personality *before* the discovery of cancer), which is largely repressed

—a person who at a young age experienced feelings of isolation, neglect, and despair in interpersonal relationships. In early adulthood, the patient then established a strong, meaningful relationship or found fulfillment in a vocation in which a great amount of energy was invested. Then, later, this relationship was lost or removed (through death, loss of child, retirement, and so forth) and the despair of childhood returned.

LeShan found that 76 percent of the 500 patients in his studies shared this basic personality profile. Interestingly enough, these people were often regarded with admiration by their friends and acquaintances because they so stoically and uncomplainingly seemed to bear great hardship and siappointment.

The Chicago Institute for Psychoanalysis conducted a ten-year study to determine if there were personality profiles for seven common psychosomatic diseases: duodenal ulcers, ulcerative colitis, bronchial asthma, hypertension, neurodermatitis (skin disorders), arthiritis, and thyrotoxicosis (overfunctioning of the thyroid). In each disease classification a personality type more likely to contract these specific disease was discovered.

In a similar manner, Doctors Meyer Friedman and Ray Rosenman, cardiologists at Mount Zion Hospital in San Francisco, discovered that there are specific personality types that predispose a person to become a cardiac patient. Their findings were published in a book that received wide acceptance: *Type A Behavior and Your Heart.*

Actually, LeShan's findings seem to confirm concepts that have appeared in medical literature for the past two thousand years. The linking of cancer and emotional states is hardly a new idea. In the second century A.D., the physician Galen observed that cheerful women were less prone to cancer than those who were depressed. Dr. Carl Simonton has traced similar expressions through medical literature to the present time—not in research, but in physicians' observations of their experience with cancer patients. He discovered that LeShan's research was also preceded by Dr. Elida Evans, a Jungian analyst, who in 1926 wrote *A Psychological Study of Cancer,* with conclusions similar to LeShan's.

Since LeShan's findings have appeared, other researchers, including Doctors A. H. Schmale, H. Iker, W. A. Greene, and D. M. Kissen, have published studies confirming LeShan's work. In 1957, Dr. Bruno Klopfer, a clinical psychologist and late president of the Society for Projective Techniques, conducted a study of cancer patients to see whether by using the Rorschach (ink blot) test he could successfully predict which patients would have fast-growing or slow-growing tumors. The results of the predictions were surprisingly successful and Dr. Klopfer interpreted them to indicate that a person with an insecure ego spent most of his (or her) energy holding himself together, with little or nothing left over to fight disease. The person with the secure ego appeared to have sufficient strength to deal with his disease.

In 1959 Dr. Eugene Pendergrass, one of America's leading radiologists and then president of the American Cancer Society, made a strong plea for a wholistic approach to the treatment of cancer:

> There is solid evidence that the course of the disease [cancer] in general is affected by emotional distress. . . . Thus, we as doctors may begin to emphasize treatment of the patient as a whole as well as the disease from which the patient is suffering. . . . As we go forward . . . searching for new means of controling growth both within the cell and through systemic influences it is my sincere hope that we can widen the quest to include the distinct possibility that within one's mind is a power capable of exerting forces which can either enhance or inhibit the progress of this disease.

Valere and I had an opportunity to meet Dr. Pendergrass and have dinner with him a few months before his death in 1980. He not only was enthusiastic about our telling Valere's story through this book, but also seemed even more convinced of the relevance of emotional factors in both contracting and fighting cancer.

Inasmuch as we knew Dr. LeShan, were impressed by his work, and were ourselves convinced of the mind/body/spirit relationship, we spent hours tracing parallels between the cancer personality profile and Valere's own personality configuration. These included extreme sensitivity and insecurity in personal relationships as a child; a nineteen-year marriage to a chronic alcoholic with intense amounts of despair and anger buried beneath a facade of calm, unruffled competence; and the subsequent break-up of that marriage, which only intensified and further buried her negative emotions. People tended to admire the way she seemed to handle all this, saying, "How do you do it?" In retrospect, it appears that she didn't.

Part of our posttherapy prevention program has involved intensive work in helping Valere to learn to express anger in a constructive manner. It sounds easier than it is, but we believe she has made considerable progress along these lines. Even if some day someone proves that there is absolutely no link between extensive repressed anger and cancer (something we frankly don't expect will happen), the other benefits she and we will have enjoyed as a result will have made the effort more than worthwhile.

Those who have experienced cancer or are in a high-risk category might do well to add constructive stress-management and personality analysis to their prevention program. (See the Suggested Reading list.)

The Simonton approach, with its emphasis on the patient's participation in the contraction and treatment of his or her disease has drawn heavy criticism on the grounds that it inflicts a burden of unnecessary and devastating guilt on the patient. In our experience, people are shaken and undone when confronted with the idea that they share some responsibility for their cancers. Some angrily refuse to consider this as a possibility. One woman became hostile when I tried to help her see that her cancer might in some way be linked to her unresolved guilt (undeserved, as I tried to point out) in relation to her daughter's suicide, despite the fact that both friends and even members of her family had come to the same conclusion. In this case, however, I am certain that the problem lay not with the concept, but with both my failure to interpret it clearly and her own refusal to let go of her guilt over the suicide. Strangely, she seemed to prefer to think that she was responsible for her own daughter's death, rather than for her own.

It seems to me that the criticisms of the "responsibility" concept in wholistic health are largely unjustified. Healing almost always involves pain of some kind. I do not feel that physical pain is any more justified than emotional pain. Furthermore, I believe that the only way to escape the burden of guilt in a healthy manner is to deal with it and dispose of it. In addition, in my experience as a counselor and pastor I have witnessed many times that emotional and physical healing are dependent upon accepting responsibility. Finally, if the concept of responsibility is skillfully interpreted, it will not be perceived as a load of guilt, but as an opportunity to make necessary changes in a person's inner life.

A recent three-year study by Professors Smith and Sebastian, two Texas A&M researchers, has revealed that there is a dramatic difference between the number of "critical incidences" in the lives of cancer patients and noncancer patients. These studies have implied a correlation between emotional history and the function of the body's immune system, as well as a critical tie between hormonal imbalance and emotional stress.

Psychological and spiritual therapy may prove to be among some of the most important weapons in the battle against cancer.

Preventive Surgery

Recently, one of Valere's clients confessed that she was on her way to an East Coast hospital to have both her breasts removed by subcutaneous mastectomy, to be followed by breast reconstruction.

"Both breasts!" Valere gasped.

"Yes," replied the woman, "my doctor says that, with my mother and my sister both having had breast cancer, I'm in a very high risk category."

This was our introduction to the practice of preventive mastectomies and breast reconstruction on the grounds of high risk. The rationale behind this seemingly extreme solution to the risk of breast cancer is the frustration doctors feel in not being able to detect cancer of the breast early enough to make a difference in the survival rate. "We wouldn't consider doing this operation at all, if we had better detecting methods," says Dr. Charles S. Rogers, a Bay City, Michigan surgeon who has performed 109 of them. "The truth is," he says, "we don't detect cancer early enough."

This practice is also based upon the statistical fact that an American woman who has had a mother with breast cancer has a one-in-five chance of contracting the disease as compared with a one-in-eleven chance. If the woman's sister also has contracted breast cancer, the risk is even higher. Another statistic that the breast reconstruction surgeons raise is that, when they have performed preventive breast mastectomies, one in ten women upon whom the operation has been performed have shown in their biopsy a cancerous or precancerous condition. Dr. Rogers also defends his surgery, maintaining that "the problem with breast removal is emotional, not rational. It has to do with the main function of the breast, and that's sex as most people see it." I think the good doctor has a rather limited—and possibly chauvinistic—view of the meaning and function of the female breast, We find it hard to accept preventive breast surgery as a justifiable preventive measure, at least on the grounds of high risk.

Apparently we're not entirely alone in that conviction. Dr. John N. Wolfe, chief of radiology at Hutzel Hospital in Detroit, says: "I have problems with it." For every surgeon who is an advocate, he continued, at least a hundred workers in cancer research are against the operation.

"It's not like having a wisdom tooth out; you've got to think about this one."

Preventive mastectomies as prophylactic measures against breast cancer on the basis of high risk may some day prove to be justifiable. Medical friends assure us that this a reasonable medical strategy. But it seems no more reasonable to us than suggesting amputation for men who have a family history of penile cancer.

Self-Examination

We've saved this one until last, trusting that all that has preceded it in our survey of preventive steps will have given added emphasis to its importance. Breast cancer is most easily cured when discovered at an early stage. Women, themselves, are the ones who stand the best chance of discovering their own early-stage cancers.

Why is it, then, that so many women still fail to conduct this simply monthly procedure which takes less than five minutes?

Until there are definitive studies indicating otherwise, we believe one of the most important reasons why women do not avail themselves of this no-cost preventive measure is their fear of finding a lump which may be cancerous. What these women need to remember is that:

seventy-five percent of American women will not be stricken with breast cancer!

eight out of ten lumps discovered in the breast are not cancerous!

the cure rate for Stage I breast cancers is better than 80 percent.

To that, add our conviction that, even if you have a Stage I or II breast cancer, you do not have to lose your breast if you choose radiation therapy—and without any lessening of your chances for survival.

Self-examination can save both your breast and your life. Why take the risk with either when it is obvious that an ounce of prevention is worth many, many pounds of cure—any cure.

11. Dispelling the Myths

In preparing this book we have been dealing with facts, people's interpretations of the facts, theories, and myths—categories which are not necessarily mutually exclusive. We have found that there is a relatively small core of fact, a fair number of theories, lots more interpretations of facts (sometimes passed off as facts) and an equal number of myths. Unfortunately—or fortunately, depending upon your point of view—today's facts can easily become tomorrow's myths.

Still, at the present time, these are some of the facts that we are dealing with in the consideration of breast cancer:

> Eighty percent of all the lumps found in women's breasts are *not* cancerous.
>
> One out of seven cancer patients is a breast cancer patient.
>
> With the exclusion of skin cancers, breast cancer is the most common malignancy in women.

One out of ten patients who die of cancer are women who have been unsuccessfully treated for breast cancer

The mortality rate for breast cancer has not been significantly reduced for the past thirty years

The rate of incidence of breast cancer in the United States has not changed since 1939

Ninety percent of all breast cancers are initially discovered by women themselves

Mammography can detect 45 percent of breast cancers not detected by the physician's manual examination

The rate of cure for minimal tumors discovered by mammography is better than 95 percent

One breast cancer out of one thousand will be healed without treatment

Stage 0 (in situ/noninvasive) breast tumors have an almost 100 percent rate of cure

Stage I breast tumors are being treated with a survival rate of better than 90 percent for five years, and better than 80 percent for ten years

Stage II breast tumors are being treated with a survival rate of 77 percent for five years and 54 percent for ten years

In 1980 10 percent of all breast tumors were Stage 0

In 1980 57 percent were Stage II tumors

In 1981 about 111,000 women were diagnosed as having breast cancer

Only 7 percent of American women contract breast cancer

Ninety-three percent of American women will *not* get breast cancer

So if you contract breast cancer, what are your chances for cure?

One of the myths that needs dispelling surrounds the term *cure*, at least so far as breast cancer is concerned. It has been customary in the medical profession to speak of cancer being "cured" when the patient has survived at least five years without a recurrence after the therapy. This led many people to assume that there was no danger of recurrence of their disease once they passed the five-year mark. This is an unfortunate misconception, for breast cancer can and sometimes does recur in "cured" breast cancer patients ten, fifteen, and even twenty years after the initial treatment. That is why we believe and recommend that a breast cancer patient who appears to have been treated successfully needs to think in terms of prevention.

Many physicians today are using a terminology that, if not as comforting as formerly, is certainly more accurate. They will usually cite three sets of data: the *recurrence rate*, representing the percentage of patients who develop another breast cancer at some time following the initial treatment; the *survival rate*, indicating the percentage of treated patients still alive five and ten years after their therapy; a *disease-free rate*, the percentage of surviving patients in whom no cancer has recurred. Obviously, the disease-free rate may be anticipated to be somewhat lower than the survival rate.

When a patient who has been treated for breast cancer has a recurrence of the disease, the physician calls this a failure. But that doesn't mean the breast cancer was not properly treated—although it can. It may mean that the conditions that gave rise to the first cancer have also given rise to another. Initially, the medical profession concentrated on treating the breast cancer itself. In recent years, there has been a recognition that sometimes the disease has metastasized and therefore needs to be treated at a distant site as well. Perhaps no great improvement in statistics can be achieved until the profession gives adequate consideration to treating the causes of cancer themselves, whatever they may prove to be.

What are the causes of cancer? As we saw in chapter ten, we still cannot answer that question with great accuracy and certainty. We do know that cancer is not one disease but many. The causes of breast cancer will probably prove to be quite different from the causes of skin cancer. Actually, we know that breast cancer itself is not one disease, but perhaps as many as fifteen different diseases, each of them caused by a varied complex of factors. Few, if any, cancers have a simple, single cause.

We have reviewed the evidence that suggests that certain carcinogens may cause breast cancer—although no carcinogen has thus been identified to date. We have reviewed means of improving the body's immune system, specifically various means of strengthening it in resisting possible viruses that induce cancer—although to date no virus in human beings has so been isolated and identified. We have considered the role that heredity may play, as well as radiation, hormones, diet, emotional factors, and stress.

Perhaps it is helpful for us to think of the onset of breast cancer in the way that Dr. Hans Selye speaks of the effect of stress as a trigger of disease. "In the body," he says, "as in the chain, the weakest link breaks down under stress although all parts are equally exposed to it. Thus, two people exposed to the same stressors may respond quite differently. How they will respond, how they will become ill, will depend upon the weakest link or links in their own bodies, and this weakness or vulnerability may be determined by a host of factors including genetic predisposition to certain diseases, environmental factors, dietary habits, exposure to carcinogens, endocrinological imbalances or changes, past medical history leaving them with vulnerabilities, personal habits and lifestyles, exposure to viruses and bacteria, as well as the strength and vitality of their immune systems.

Therefore, it is time to dispel the popular myth which causes us to look for but one cause of cancer, while at the same time attempting to discover the one cure for it. There is no single arch villain that we can pinpoint.

Another myth which must be dispelled is the cavalier assumption that a woman's breast is a readily expendable part of the anatomy with little value beyond the cosmetic. The breasts are part of her visible womanhood. A man can live without his penis and scrotum, his visible manhood, but he ought not to have to do so unless it is absolutely necessary. Neither should a woman have to give up her breasts without real justification, particularly when the medical profession is divided on that very issue.

A woman's breasts are part of her beauty. Men have been telling her so since the beginning of time. Nor is it frivolous for her to regard her breasts as a very important part of her sexual self, something that men have also confirmed in the way they relate to her.

Dr. Jerzy Einhorn, Director of the Department of Nonsurgical Oncology at the Karolinska Hospital and Institute in Stockholm, Sweden, says that he had always believed that he was sympathetic to the feelings of women breast cancer patients. Then one day a psychologist in the Karolinska Hospital came to him with a proposal to study twenty mastectomy patients, to examine their feelings and perceptions before and after their surgery. The interviews would be taped and held confidential. Dr. Einhorn agreed to the study. Two years later he listened to the conversations that had been recorded on tape. "I was shocked when I heard what my patients felt about having a mastectomy. I don't know if a physician can understand what it means to get a diagnosis of a disease as feared as breast cancer if you haven't gone through it yourself." The anger the women expressed both toward their operation and him left an indelible impression upon him. The physician may never know how a woman feels on this score, but he can at least be aware that he cannot know.

In a survey of more than 2,000 women across the United States, the National Cancer Institute found that when asked their first impressions about breast cancer, women mentioned "loss of breast" three times more frequently than anything else. The report said that this underscores the powerful psychological impact of breast cancer through its association with surgical treatment. The time has come to dispel the myth that a diagnosis of breast cancer equals the loss of a breast.

We think it is time for surgeons to stop misleading women into believing that their security depends upon the amount of surgery performed. "How can you be sure you got it all with a lumpectomy?" a surgeon asked me a few months ago. "Your wife will never feel secure," he added. His concept of security depended upon Dr. Halsted's erroneous assumptions about how breast cancer spreads.

What we are protesting is not surgery in general or surgery for breast cancer in particular, but the precipitate rush to surgery that characterizes the experience of far too many women today. Dr. Norman Shealy of LaCrosse, Wisconsin, himself a surgeon, once told me of a study of 250 patients who had undergone surgery for a ruptured disc. Of this group, 6 were discovered to have actually had a ruptured disc, 42 were questionable, and 202 did not. I realize that it's not very scientific to draw parallels between these two unrelated types of surgery, but I cannot escape the conviction that just as preachers feel impelled to preach (often, perhaps, without justification), so surgeons feel obligated to cut. We're not alone in feeling somewhat uneasy about the prevalence of surgery in this country.

Any part of the body can be sacrificed when it is imperative to do so. But we are convinced that the sacrifice ought not to be any greater than the risk. Organ preservation, when it is possible, ought to have a higher priority. Many of us can remember when it was thought essential to remove tonsils and adenoids as standard operating procedure. Today, if they can be preserved, they are not removed. At the 1980 panel discussion under the auspices of the American College of Radiology, Dr. Einhorn outlined some of the important advances in organ preservation which we are making today:

> What organs can we preserve today? Well, we preserve the eye by radiotherapy and the vision in retinaoblastomas. We preserve the penis in treatment by radiotherapy of penile cancer (not very often seen in our country—it's more common in the United States). We can preserve the breast of the woman, if the tumor is not too large. In laryngeal carcinoma (cancer of the larynx), we can preserve the vocal cords and the larynx by radiotherapy. In some situations, in carcinoma of the bladder, we can preserve that organ, too.

Cancer is no longer synonymous with loss of the organ. The greatest conflict in the treatment of breast cancer today is obviously between the rival claims of the surgeons and the radiologists. Unlike many segments of American life, one of these does not have to be victorious at the expense of the other. One of the contestants does not have to be driven from the field. Attempts by some segments of the medical profession to paper over this important controversy are a disservice to both groups as well as the public. There is a dramatic disagreement between these two branches of medicine and the public deserves to have a better view of the issues involved.

The surgeons can point to almost a century of experience and data and say with justification: we've proven what the mastectomy can do. The radiologists come along with their own statistics that indicate they can meet the challenge of Stage I and II breast cancers with results as good or better. Surgeons counter with the charge that these studies are biased in the selection of patients for the studies and have not covered a sufficient amount of time to see if the reported results stand up. This is rebutted by Dr. Bernard Fisher of the University of Pittsburgh, who points out that since the vast majority of treatment failures occur within the first three years after the initial therapy, the probability that any major differences will have developed by the end of ten or fifteen years is extremely unlikely.

Some surgeons point to the study published in 1972 by Dr. H.J.B. Atkins at Guy's Hospital, London, as proof that the radiation approach is less successful than mastectomy. These studies have been flashed at me more than a few times in discussions with surgeons. My response has been and continues to be that to use those studies as "proof" is patently dishonest at worst and unprofessional at best. The Atkins studies and results were based upon radiation doses that were totally inadequate by current standards—3,500 to 3,800 rads to the breast and 2,500 to 2,700 rads to the nodes. That is not what is being offered to breast cancer patients today and it is irresponsible to leave the patient with that impression.

If the surgeons are critical of the patient selection for the radiation studies, radiologists are no less critical of some of the results attributed to the mastectomy. Dr. Luther Brady cautions: "You also have to remember that 80 percent of all the patients in this country with cancer of the breast are operated upon in hospitals of 250 beds or less by surgeons who do one, two, or three cases per year. How can you expect under those circumstances to maintain clinical competence, or understanding, or even skill, when you don't work any more often on breast cancer than once a year?" Furthermore, points out Dr. Brady, at a time when more and more surgeons are turning toward the less radical mastectomies, too few have sufficient experience in the less radical procedure. "As a result," he says, "we're now seeing an increasingly greater frequency of local recurrences because of inappropriate selection criteria for the operation and the skills that are not honed to the point of doing it properly."

In response to the oft-quoted argument by surgeons that only the mastectomy can deal with the multicentricity of cancer (additional cancer sites) often found in the breast, radiologists counter that studies indicate that radiation handles these just as successfully.

Dr. Moses, our surgeon in Dallas, warned us that Valere would be "horribly mutilated" if she submitted to radiation therapy. He had seen scores of women permanently disfigured by radiation treatment of the breast. Imputing the very best of motives to Dr. Moses' statement, I can only assume that he was referring to the sometimes disfiguring results that accompanied the early use of radiation therapy. But that is like remembering the days in which surgery was performed by barbers, for the technology of radiation of the breast has improved tremendously since the days when the old X-ray machines were used and healthy as well as cancerous tissues were damaged and destroyed. Surely every surgeon knows that the breast radiology of today is entirely different from the treatment available thirty years ago. Today the radiologist can select a suitable ray—beta, alpha, or gamma—and direct the ray at a small area, near the surface or deep within the body, irradiating either the whole breast or an area of half an inch. In doing so, he can deliver exact, controlled doses and at the same time spare the chest wall and the lungs. Different rays are used for different needs and by bombarding the cancer from several different directions, he can minimize the dosage to healthy cells nearby. In short, radiology today is a precise technology that is becoming ever more precise.

Dr. Jerzy Einhorn believes mounting evidence indicates breast irradiation "does more than cure cancer. With surgery the bulk of the tumor is removed and thrown away. With radiotherapy, the damaged tissue is left *in loco* [in place] to be absorbed, and this boosts the immunological reactivity of the host [the body irradiated]. . . . Most of the results of studies done using irradiated tumor cells injected in animals or even in humans indicates that the effect of radiotherapy is very beneficial to the host. I personally believe that some of the good results we get with radiotherapy depends upon this boosting effect."

Dr. Brady believes that when the lumpectomy and 5,000 rads over five weeks are boosted with an additional, highly concentrated dosage either by electron beam or implants (which is what Valere received), the problem of recurrence of cancer in the breast is virtually eliminated. "We have no local recurrences in our patients in the lumpectomy site by this treatment." He estimates that 60,000 of the 111,000 women estimated as contracting breast cancer in 1981 could do as well without mastectomy as with it.

But the controversy rages on and many women won't even realize they have a choice. Why? Because the radiation alternative has not been getting a fair hearing. Patients are referred directly from their physicians to a surgeon. Rarely do physicians recommend seeing a radiation oncologist too. All too often, they have not kept up with developments in the field and they have tended to take the word of the surgeons that radiation for breast cancer is dangerous, new, and untried.

Furthermore, the American Cancer Society up to the present has almost entirely represented the surgeon's point of view. For example, several years ago the society put on a program for the American College of Obstetrics and Gynecology, related to cancer of the breast. There were four speakers on the panel, all surgeons. There were no diagnostic radiologists, no medical oncologists, and no radiation therapists. Is it any wonder that obstetricians and gynecologists are often so poorly informed or prejudiced in the direction of surgery?

During the preparation of this book, we telephoned and visited various local American Cancer Society offices to speak with their representatives and examine the literature available without cost to the public. With little exception the literature and advice have remained pretty much the same: mastectomy is the only recommended therapy. Referrals were made to surgeons, never to radiologists. In Santa Fe, New Mexico, in mid-1981, for example, when we persisted in asking about radiation as an alternative therapy for Stage I and II breast cancers, we were referred to a local surgeon for more information. In all visits to an ACS center, we were given the previously mentioned booklet by Dr. Phillip Strax, *Breast Cancer is Curable,* in which the author states: "At this time, surgery is the most effective treatment for breast cancer." Although Dr. Strax acknowledges that the treatment of breast cancer "must tend to involve differences of opinion," he does not mention irradiation.

When this manuscript was in final draft, we decided to make one last visit to a local ACS office. Valere called the American Cancer Society number listed for a city in Pennsylvania, and said that she was calling to procure information for a friend whose physician had detected a suspicious lump. "I'd like to come by your office and pick up some literature, if I might," Valere told the representative.

"Well, I suppose so," said the woman.

"Do you have some materials on the various alternative treatments?" Valere asked.

"Of course not," replied the woman somewhat indignantly. "Your friend will get all that information from her surgeon. She does have a surgeon, doesn't she?"

"Not yet," Valere replied.

"Well," continued the woman, "we couldn't do anything like that. We have lots of information here, but it's for professionals only. I couldn't give it to you." She went on to recommend a local surgeon, and said Valere could stop by the office for the printed materials available for the lay person.

When Valere returned from that ACS office, she had been given "Breast Cancer is Curable" by Dr. Strax (printed in 1975); a pamphlet, "Cancer Facts For Women"; a booklet of statistics, "Cancer Facts and Figures, 1981"; "How to Examine Your Breasts," a breast self-examination quiz; and a booklet, "Facts on Breast Cancer," all published by the ACS. Only in the latter was there a noticeable change in ACS advice. The Treatment section begins with: "Although surgery is the most effective method of treating most women with breast cancer, radiation therapy and chemotherapy, in combination with surgery, are being used with increasing frequency."

After this introduction, there is a long paragraph on surgery, followed by a section under the heading, Radiation Therapy, explaining how radiation works on cancer cells, how it is used in combination with other treatment methods, and a listing of radiation's side effects: "skin reactions, nausea, vomiting, and a feeling of tiredness." No mention is made of the side effects of the mastectomy, nor is there any suggestion that breast irradiation may be considered as an alternative to the mastectomy. A full page is given to rehabilitation, one brief paragraph to the biopsy, and no mention is made of the two-step procedure in diagnosis.

In our opinion, this pamphlet, published in 1978 and revised in 1980, still withholds essential information that should be available to every woman.

It appears that the American Cancer Society is still pretty much under the influence and control of the surgeons, most of whom seem to vigorously resist acknowledging radiation as an alternative, let alone the right of the women to participate in choosing from among alternatives.

Why are so many surgeons still so resistant? Some critics, Dr. George Crile, Jr., among them, have charged that it is a matter of economics. Crile says, "A judge whose salary and reputation depended upon whether the verdict was for plaintiff or defendent, prosecutor or prisoner, would be as little trusted as a general in the pay of the enemy." It is difficult to be objective—even among scientists—when large amounts of money are dependent upon a controversial procedure. But that is hardly a phenomenon unique to surgeons. Who among us is not unconsciously motivated in our work or profession by economics?

I think Rose Kushner is closer to the mark when she cites the training of the surgeon. As Kushner puts it, "Surgeons, after all, are trained to think of surgical solutions to the problems of disease. . . . To stop a century-old procedure in favor of one they have struggled against so long and so vehemently would be an admission that they have been wrong." What professional likes to admit he or she may have been wrong?

Dr. Crile believes the change in physicians' attitudes, at least in part, will have to come from the medical schools themselves. "It is hard enough to change the mind of a student about some belief that he has accepted, but it is nearly impossible to change the mind of a teacher in respect to a subject he has been teaching."

Equally difficult to change, it seems, is the stance of the American Cancer Society. We have been critical of the ACS because we feel that the help it provided us—principally information—was minimal. We would not have learned that there was a radiation therapy alternative if our only source of information had been ACS. Millions of Americans who contribute to that society do not realize that they are financing a very one-sided approach to breast cancer. Programs that promote emphasis on early detection of breast cancer through self-examination and the Reach to Recovery program are excellent, but I think we have a right to expect something more of ACS. As Dr. Crile says, "Much good is being done by the American Cancer Society's Reach to Recovery program, designed to rehabilitate women after mastectomies. But would it not be wiser for the Society to use its influence to prevent the injuries rather than to compensate for them?" We think so.

Many surgeons have also resisted the issue of informed choice and patient participation in the choice of therapy, as well as the use of the two-step approach that divides the biopsy from the therapy. And, if the American Cancer Society hasn't exactly opposed these things, neither has it led the way in championing them. Some of the surgeons with whom we've spoken now have come to accept these ideas—but grudgingly. Many of them find it unacceptable for patients to assume responsibility for their own medical therapy (a reaction which is not unique to surgeons).

The purpose of this book is not to do battle with the surgeons, but it is to do battle with the kind of arrogance that can only hurt the profession in the long run, not to mention their patients. As reported by the *Dallas Times Herald,* a women who tried to make an appointment with a surgeon for a second opinion regarding her breast cancer, was flatly refused. The surgeon told her, "I would be dead in this city if I took one of Dr. X's patients." Should the ego of the physician be more important than the welfare of the patient?

The tactics of intimidation we encountered with Dr. Moses have been experienced by other breast cancer patients who have expressed an interest in treatment other than mastectomy. When interviewed by a Dallas journalist in December, 1980, Dr. Dale Fuller, a Dallas radiologist, said, "There are surgeons here who, *if demanded by the patient,* (italics mine) will do a lumpectomy (to be followed by radiation therapy) if the patient will listen to all of the reasons why she shouldn't (make that choice)."

In an August 17, 1981 conversation with us, however, Dr. Fuller reports that since he made that statement a "very pleasant change has begun to take place" in the Dallas area. Although some surgeons are still strongly opposed, Dr. Fuller has found an increasing number who are making fair presentations of the alternative treatments to their patients. In some cases, Dr. Fuller said, the surgeons themselves have set up consultations for the patient with radiologists and medical oncologists. To be sure, these may be at the request of the patient, but Dr. Fuller feels this is a welcome change, regardless who initiates it. Actually, says Dr. Fuller, it is the new awareness of the patient that is helping to bring about this change. The strong opposition which he noted less than a year ago has begun to crumble because of the attention this subject has received both in the lay press and medical publications.

There are other signs of hope as well. Dr. Charles R. Smart, the American College of Surgeons' assistant director for cancer, was recently quoted in *Medical World News* concerning the mounting evidence for the effective results from lumpectomy plus irradiation, as saying: "If the numbers hold up on these studies, it would mean a whole new ball game—that there is some validity to this alternative method."

Dr. Jerzy Einhorn says that in Sweden a breast cancer patient is handled by a team approach. If the diagnosis indicates the possibility of a breast malignancy, appointments are made for her with both a surgeon and a radiologist. After that, she is taken to another room where, with the assistance of a nurse who is specially trained, she makes her own decision.

Dr. Luther W. Brady has called for the same kind of interdisciplinary approach in the United States: "We must eliminate chauvinism about our specialities and determine how we can best coordinate surgery, radiation therapy, and chemotherapy to optimize treatment. . . . Only by a modulated, multidisciplinary approach can the cure rate for breast cancer be significantly advanced." That's what we're asking for—not the victory of the good guys vs the bad guys, but the kind of co-operation that ensures that the real winner will be the patient.

May we expect that co-operative team approach here? Tentatively, our answer is: Yes, but don't hold your breath; it won't happen over the weekend.

Even so, there are encouraging signs. For instance, Dr. William Feller, associate professor of surgery at Georgetown Hospital, told us that he believes it is absolutely necessary to discuss fairly the available alternative treatments when a woman is diagnosed with breast cancer: "The patient has a right to an informed choice." He said that most doctors today, when it comes to the best treatment for breast cancer, do not believe the final answer is in. "I present irradiation as an acceptable method," he says, "but we do not have sufficient long-term data to designate one method as a clear first choice. Perhaps by 1985 we may have enough data to be more certain. Present data looks good, but we need a lot more." In the meantime, Dr. Feller explains to each patient the alternatives open to her, and approximately 20 percent of his patients elect removal of the tumor and irradiation. Most of these treatments are performed at Georgetown University Hospital. Dr. Feller does not, however, abandon the patient who fails to take his advice. "It's not 'I'm the big doctor and you do what I say or else!' " He believes that the physician must acknowledge the dignity of his patient.

Another prominent surgeon, Dr. Caldwell Esselstyn, chief breast surgeon at the Cleveland Clinic in Ohio, acknowledges that 90 percent of those with operable breast cancer are candidates for local excision (removal of the tumor) plus irradiation. "More and more," says Dr. Esselstyn, "we're learning that ultimate survival is determined not by the quantity of flesh removed, but by the aggressiveness of the cancer in the particular individual."

Another surgeon, Dr. Richard Bassin of New York, told us in August, 1981, that he believed most surgeons were not well informed about the results being achieved with breast irradiation in combination with the lumpectomy. "Many of us just are not getting the data," he said. When he was asked to write an article on the subject, Dr. Bassin looked for irradiation data and was surprised with what he found. Today, therefore, he is more disposed to the consideration of irradiation as a viable alternative in early-stage breast cancer. He believes more surgeons are changing their attitudes because trial results are becoming more available.

"There's been a definite change in attitudes on this subject in Massachusetts in the last few years," Dr. William D. Bloomer told us in August, 1981. Dr. Bloomer, who is associate professor of radiotherapy at Harvard Medical School, says that even "older surgeons in the state are less recalcitrant to offer radiation" as an alternative. When we asked whether this change was in any way a result of the recent Massachusetts law mandating that physicians outline alternative treatments to all breast cancer patients, Dr. Bloomer laughed and said, "Well, no one's going to want to admit that, but it has got to be a factor. After all," he continued, "the threat of being sued is a rather considerable motivation." In addition, Dr. Bloomer believes that general surgeons now in training are seeing that irradiation produces a better cosmetic result and this will eventually affect practices in hospitals throughout the country. He feels that although there are some cases in which the mastectomy may be justified—such as in patients whose tumor is diffused throughout the breast—the mastectomy will be used less and less in the years ahead. He is encouraged, he said, because even obstetricians and gynecologists are beginning to refer patients to radiotherapists.

The final myth that needs to be dispelled relates to the

pervasive gloom that usually settles over the subject of breast cancer. We believe this is a time for hope.

As already indicated, one source of hope is the opportunity for women to preserve their breasts in Stage I and II breast cancers through the combined use of lumpectomy and irradiation. Also promising are the advances taking place in radiation and chemotherapeutic technology. In chapter eight we outlined some experimental therapies that in the years ahead may make the treatment of breast cancer even more optimistic. We have heard of four or five different testing procedures which could help to detect breast cancer in women on the basis of regular screening, both more accurately and earlier than the mammogram. We discussed these with American Cancer Society vice president Arthur Holleb in April, 1981, and he said that although all are presently experimental, he had high hopes for several of the techniques—but only after sufficient time for accurate testing.

So we must begin to dispel the myth of hopelessness that has accumulated around breast cancer. Even breast cancer that has metastasized to the lungs or liver should not be regarded as a hopeless situation. As Dr. George Crile has said, "Cancer obeys no laws, not even its own."

One surgeon, when it was apparent that we were not persuading him and he was not influencing us, said: "I hope you don't have to regret this decision in five or ten years. Then it would be too late to realize your mistake." But he was wrong in his reasoning. For even if Valere should become a victim of cancer at some future date, it would not mean that we had made the wrong choice. Many women choose mastectomy and still die of cancer. That does not make their choice "wrong." As that surgeon surely knows, when a breast cancer patient who has been treated either with mastectomy or irradiation later contracts another cancer, it is seldom because of the failure of the treatment to the breast, but because the breast cancer metastasized to another part of the body *before* the breast was treated. Neither mastectomy nor irradiation have failed when that occurs. The underlying problem still must be solved by medicine.

We are confident that we made the right choice. There is no reason to believe we will ever feel differently about that choice.

We began this book in anxiety, wanting desperately that women take responsibility for knowing all they can about this subject and for preparing themselves to make responsible choices. We close it in hope, convinced that women have a better chance than ever before to meet and prevail over this disease.

However, this new hope will not be placed in your hands, nor will it be delivered with the morning newspaper. If you want it, you will at least need to do the following to bring it about:

- First of all, take responsibility for your own body; don't expect or let someone else do it for you.
- Keep yourself well informed.
- Examine your own breasts on a monthly basis.
- Know and observe the danger signals and seek professional help as soon as you detect anything which is suspicious.
- Make certain you will not be rushed into surgery you don't want if through a mammogram or other diagnostic tool it is determined that you may have breast cancer.
- Make your choice for a therapy on the basis of as much information as you can get if you are diagnosed as having breast cancer.
- Take responsibility if you are treated for breast cancer, for doing all that you can to avoid a recurrence, using the best information that is available to you from different disciplines.

So, to you, the women throughout the nation, we say: you have the right and the power—exercise both.

And to the physicians of this country, we close with a gentle reminder from Hippocrates that will be familiar, if not always well remembered:

Primum non nocere.
First of all, do no harm.

Suggested Reading

Achterberg, Jeanne and Lawlis, G. Frank. *Bridges of the Bodymind.* Champaign, Illinois: Institute of Personality and Ability Testing, 1980.

———. *Imagery of Cancer.* Champaign, Illinois: Institute of Personality and Ability Testing, 1978.

Althouse, Lawrence W. *Rediscovering the Gift of Healing.* Nashville: Abingdon Press, 1977.

Benson, Herbert. *The Relaxation Response.* New York: Avon Books, 1978.

———. *The Mind/Body Effect.* New York: Berkeley Books, 1980.

Brody, Jane. *Jane Brody's Nutrition Book.* New York: W.W. Norton & Company, Inc., 1981.

Brody, Jane, and Holleb, Arthur. *You Can Fight Cancer and Win.* New York: Quadrangle, 1977.

Cope, Oliver. *The Breast: A Health Guide for Women of All Ages.* Boston: Houghton Mifflin Co., 1974.

Cousins, Norman. *Anatomy of an Illness as Perceived by the Patient: Reflections on Healing and Regeneration.* New York: W.W. Norton & Company, Inc., 1979.

Crile, George, Jr. *What Women Should Know about the Breast Cancer Controversy.* New York: Pocket Books, 1974.

Fredericks, Carleton. *Winning the Fight Against Breast Cancer, The Nutritional Approach.* New York: Grosset & Dunlap, 1977.

Green, Elmer, and Green, Alyce. *Beyond Bio-Feedback.* New York: Delacorte Press, 1977

Hutschnecker, Arnold. *The Will to Happiness.* New York: Cornerstone Library, 1972.

———. *The Will To Live.* New York: Cornerstone Library, 1974.

Kushner, Rose. *Why Me?* New York: New American Library, 1975

LeShan, Lawrence. *You Can Fight For Your Life.* New York: Jove, 1978

Morra, Marion, and Potts, Eva. *Choices: Realistic Alternatives in Cancer Treatment.* New York: Avon, 1980.

Pelletier, Kenneth. *Mind as Healer, Mind as Slayer: A Wholistic Approach to Preventing Stress Disorders.* New York: Delta, 1977.

Rollin, Betty. *First You Cry.* New York: New American Library, 1977

Selye, Hans. *Stress Without Distress.* New York: New American Library, 1974.

Simonton, O. Carl; Simonton, Stephanie Matthews-; and Creighton, James, *Getting Well Again—A Step-by-Step, Self-Help Guide to Overcoming Cancer for Patients and their Families,* J.P. Tarcher, Los Angeles, 1978.

Clinical Oncology for Medical Students and Physicians: A Multidisciplinary Approach. 1978: The University of Rochester School of Medicine and Dentistry/American Cancer Society.

For the interested reader, the following is a list of the studies mentioned in this book.

Atkins, H.; Hayward, J.L.; Klugman, D.J.; and Wayte, A.B. "Treatment of Early Breast Cancer—A Report After Ten Years of Clinical Trial." *British Medical Journal* 11:423–29, 1972.

Bedwinek, John. "Treatment of Stage I and II Andenocarcinoma of the Breast by Tumor Excision and Irradiation." Division of Radiation Oncology, Mallinckrodt Institute of Radiology, Washington University School of Medicine, (unpublished), 1981.

Bedwinek, John M.; Perez, Carol A.; Kramer, Simon; Brady, Luther; Goodman, Robert; and Grundy, Graham. "Irradiation as the Primary Management of Stage I and II Adenocarcinoma of the Breast: Analysis of the RTOG Breast Registry." *Cancer Clinical Trials* 3:000–000, 1980.

Bonadonna, Gianni; Rossi, Anna; Valagussa, Pinuccia; Banfi, Alberto; and Veronesi, Umberto. "Adjuvant Chemotherapy with CMF in Breast Cancer with Positive Axillary Nodes."

Instituto Nazionale Tumori, Milano, Italy, 1977.

Brady, Luther W. "Cancer of the Breast: A Time For Caution." *American Journal of Roentgenol* 129:969–73, December, 1977.

———. "Cancer of the Breast: Treatment Today." *Frontiers of of Radiation Therapy and Oncology* Vol. 11, 1976.

Brady, Luther W.; Einhorn, Jerzy; Wizenberg, Morris J.; Althouse, Valere F.; and Madell, Samuel H. "The Curative Treatment of Cancer: Organ Preservation through Radiotherapy," transcript of Medical X-Ray Forum, American College of Radiology, October 15, 1980.

Brady, Luther W.; Fletcher, Gilbert H.; and Levitt, Seymour. "Cancer of the Breast: The Role of Radiation Therapy after Mastectomy." *Cancer,* Vol. 39, No. 6, June, 1977.

Brown, G.S.; Kramer, S.; Brady, L.; and Tobin, D.A. "Primary Irradiation of Stage I and Stage II Adenocarcinoma of the Breast." *International Journal of Radiation Oncology Biol. Phys.* Vol. 2, 1977.

Heuson, J.C.; Leclercq, G.; and Mattheiem. "Current Strategy in Breast Cancer Treatment." *Recent Advances in Cancer Treatment,* ed. by Tagnon, H.J. and Staquet, M.J., Raven Press, New York, 1977.

Levene, Martin B. "A New Role For Radiation Therapy." *American Journal of Nursing* September, 1977, Vol. 77, No. 9.

Levene, M.B.; Harris, J.R.; and Hellman, S. "Treatment of Carcinoma of the Breast by Radiation Therapy." *Cancer* Vol. 39, No. 6, 1977.

Mustakallio, S. "Treatment of Breast Cancer by Tumor Extirpation and Roentgen Therapy Instead of Radical Operation." *Journal of Faculty Radiology* 6:23–26, 1954.

Peters, M.V. "Cutting the 'Gordian knot' in Breast Cancer." *Annual of the Royal College of Physicians and Surgeons, Canada* 8:186–92, 1975.

Peters, M.V. "Wedge Resection and Irradiation—an Effective Treatment in Early Breast Cancer." *Journal of the American Medical Association* 200:18–21, 1967.

Prosnitz, L.R.; Goldenberg, I.S.; Packard, R.A.; Levene, M.B.; Harris, J.; Hellman, S.; Wallner, P.E.; Brady, L.W.; Mansfield, C.M.; and Kramer, S. "Radiation Therapy as Initial Treatment for Early Stage Cancer of the Breast without Mastectomy." *Cancer* 39:917–23, 1977.

Rissanean, P.M. "A Combination of Conservative and Radical Surgery Combined with Radiotherapy in the Treatment of

Stage I Carcinoma of the Breast." *British Journal of Radiology* 42:423–26, 1969.
Rosata, Francis; Martin, William L.; and Brady, Luther W. "Simple Mastectomy and Radiotherapy in the Treatment of Breast Cancer." *The American Surgeon* Vol. 35, No. 9, September, 1969.
Wallner, Paul E. "Radiation Therapy in the Management of Primary Breast Cancer." *The Journal of the Pennsylvania Osteopathic Medical Association* Spring, 1975, Vol. 17, No. 2.
Wallner, Paul E.; Brady, L.W.; Loughead, J.; Matsumoto, T.; Antoniades, J.; Prasavinichai, S.; Glassburn, J.R.; Asbell, S.O.; and Damsker, J.I. "Subtotal Mastectomy and Radiation Therapy in the Definitive Management of Localized Breast Malignancy." *American Journal of Roentgenol* 127:507, 1976.
The White House Conference: *Breast Cancer: A Report To The Profession,* November 22–23, 1976, Washington, D.C.
Wise, L.; Mason, A.Y.; and Ackerman, L.V. "Local Excision and Radiation: an Alternative Method for the Treatment of Early Mammary Cancer." Annual *Surgery* 174:392–401, 1972.

Where to Get Help

If you would like further information about medical personnel and facilities in your area with experience in the combined use of radiology and lumpectomy, we suggest you contact the Radiation Oncology Study Center at 925 Chestnut Street, Philadelphia, Pennsylvania 19107. Telephone: 215–574–3150.

Index